P9-AGH-395

90

Curbside Consultation
in Pediatric Ophthalmology

49 Clinical Questions

Curbside Consultation in Pediatrics
SERIES

SERIES EDITOR, LISA B. ZAOUTIS, MD

Curbside Consultation
in Pediatric Ophthalmology

49 Clinical Questions

Editor

Rudolph S. Wagner, MD

*Clinical Professor and Director of
Pediatric Ophthalmology
Institute of Ophthalmology and Visual Science
Rutgers—New Jersey Medical School
Newark, New Jersey*

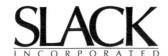

INCORPORATED

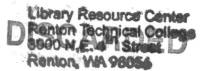

Library Resource Center
Renton Technical College
3000 N.E. 4th Street
Renton, WA 98056

www.Healio.com/books

ISBN: 978-1-61711-059-7

Copyright © 2014 by SLACK Incorporated

All rights reserved. No part of this book may be reproduced, stored in a retrieval system or transmitted in any form or by any means, electronic, mechanical, photocopying, recording or otherwise, without written permission from the publisher, except for brief quotations embodied in critical articles and reviews.

The procedures and practices described in this book should be implemented in a manner consistent with the professional standards set for the circumstances that apply in each specific situation. Every effort has been made to confirm the accuracy of the information presented and to correctly relate generally accepted practices. The authors, editor, and publisher cannot accept responsibility for errors or exclusions or for the outcome of the material presented herein. There is no expressed or implied warranty of this book or information imparted by it. Care has been taken to ensure that drug selection and dosages are in accordance with currently accepted/recommended practice. Due to continuing research, changes in government policy and regulations, and various effects of drug reactions and interactions, it is recommended that the reader carefully review all materials and literature provided for each drug, especially those that are new or not frequently used. Any review or mention of specific companies or products is not intended as an endorsement by the author or publisher.

SLACK Incorporated uses a review process to evaluate submitted material. Prior to publication, educators or clinicians provide important feedback on the content that we publish. We welcome feedback on this work.

Published by: SLACK Incorporated
                6900 Grove Road
                Thorofare, NJ 08086 USA
                Telephone: 856-848-1000
                Fax: 856-848-6091
                www.healio.com

Contact SLACK Incorporated for more information about other books in this field or about the availability of our books from distributors outside the United States.

Library of Congress Cataloging-in-Publication Data

Curbside consultation in pediatric ophthalmology : 49 clinical questions / [edited by] Rudolph S. Wagner.
    p. ; cm.
  Includes bibliographical references and index.
   ISBN 978-1-61711-059-7 (alk. paper)
  I. Wagner, Rudolph S., 1952- editor of compilation.
  [DNLM: 1. Eye Diseases--diagnosis. 2. Eye Diseases--therapy. 3. Child. 4. Infant. WW 600]
  RE48.2.C5
  618.92'0977--dc23
                        2014000789

For permission to reprint material in another publication, contact SLACK Incorporated. Authorization to photocopy items for internal, personal, or academic use is granted by SLACK Incorporated provided that the appropriate fee is paid directly to Copyright Clearance Center. Prior to photocopying items, please contact the Copyright Clearance Center at 222 Rosewood Drive, Danvers, MA 01923 USA; phone: 978-750-8400; Web site: www.copyright.com; email: info@copyright.com

Printed in the United States of America.

Last digit is print number: 10 9 8 7 6 5 4 3 2 1

618.920977 CURBSID 2014p

Curbside consultation in
pediatric ophthalmology

Dedication

This book is dedicated to my wife, Jean, and our children, Katie, Elizabeth, Julie, and Christine, and to the families of all of the contributing authors for their patience, love, and understanding.

Contents

Acknowledgments

This book was completed with the help of many of the finest ophthalmologists and people throughout the world. I purposely invited recognized experts on particular topics to contribute chapters. Having written many chapters in various textbooks, I have come to realize that matching the authors with subject matter they are passionate about is critical for the success of this type of book. Many of the authors have expressed to me the enjoyment they have in describing complicated ophthalmic conditions for their healthcare provider colleagues who are not ophthalmologists. Ophthalmologists and in particular, pediatric ophthalmologists, generally love their work and it shows. I believe the enthusiasm of the authors is expressed in their writings and I will be forever grateful to all of the contributors.

About the Editor

Rudolph S. Wagner, MD graduated from the University of Notre Dame with a BS degree and received his MD degree from Rutgers—New Jersey Medical School. He completed his Ophthalmology Residency at Rutgers—New Jersey Medical School and Fellowship in Pediatric Ophthalmology at Wills Eye Hospital of Jefferson Medical College in Philadelphia, Pennsylvania. He is presently Clinical Professor of Ophthalmology at the Institute of Ophthalmology and Visual Science of Rutgers—New Jersey Medical School in Newark, New Jersey and Director of Pediatric Ophthalmology at the same institution. He has published over 140 scientific articles and has contributed to many chapters in textbooks. He is co-editor of the *Journal of Pediatric Ophthalmology and Strabismus*. He has been teaching and practicing pediatric ophthalmology for over 25 years and has particular interests in neonatal ophthalmology and pediatric conjunctivitis. He enjoys teaching eye surgery in third world countries and most recently traveled to Ulan Baatar, Mongolia with ORBIS. In 2012 he was presented the Senior Honor Award from the American Academy of Ophthalmology (AAO) in Chicago, Illinois.

Contributing Authors

Javaneh Abbasian, MD (Question 31)
Assistant Professor of Ophthalmology
University of Illinois at Chicago
Chicago, Illinois

Ismael Al Ghamdi, MD (Question 19)
Consultant Ophthalmologist
Prince Sultan Military Medical City, Riyadh
  (PSMMC)
Kingdom of Saudi Arabia

Robert W. Arnold, MD, FAAP (Question 2)
Alaska Blind Child Discovery
Alaska Children's Eye & Strabismus, LLC
Anchorage, Alaska

Kyle Arnoldi, CO (Question 30)
Instructor in Ophthalmology
State University of New York at Buffalo
Department of Ophthalmology
Chief Orthoptist
Ira G. Ross Eye Institute
Buffalo, New York

Nicholas R Binder, MD (Question 25)
Pediatric Ophthalmology and Strabismus
  Fellow
University of Southern California
Department of Ophthalmology
Children's Hospital Los Angeles
Los Angeles, California

Kara Cavuoto, MD (Question 20)
Assistant Professor of Clinical Ophthalmology
University of Miami
Bascom Palmer Eye Institute
Miami, Florida

R.V. Paul Chan, MD, FACS (Question 39)
Associate Professor of Ophthalmology
St Giles Associate Professor of Pediatric Retina
New York-Presbyterian Hospital
Weill Cornell Medical College
New York, New York

David S. Chu, MD (Question 46)
Clinical Associate Professor
Institute of Ophthalmology & Visual Science
Rutgers - New Jersey Medical School
Newark, New Jersey

William Constad, MD (Question 12)
Clinical Professor
Rutgers Medical School
Department of Ophthalmology and Visual
  Sciences
Newark, New Jersey

*Patrick A. DeRespinis, MD, FACS, FAAP, FAAO
(Question 27)*
Director, Pediatric Ophthalmology &
  Strabismus
NS/LIJ Healthcare Systems at Staten Island
  University Hospital
Associate Clinical Professor of Ophthalmology
Rutgers University
Department of Ophthalmology
New Jersey Medical School
Newark, New Jersey

Mark Dorfman, MD (Question 20)
Managing Partner
Eye Surgery Associates
Weston, Florida

Dawn Duss, MD (Questions 5, 9)
Nemours Children's Clinic
Division of Ophthalmology
Department of Pediatric Surgery
Jacksonville, Florida

Brian J. Forbes, MD, PhD (Question 31)
Associate Professor of Ophthalmology
The Children's Hospital of Philadelphia
The Perelman School of Medicine at
  The University of Pennsylvania
Philadelphia, Pennsylvania

Larry Frohman, MD (Question 32)
Professor of Ophthalmology & Visual Sciences
& Neurology and Neurosciences
Rutgers—New Jersey Medical School
Newark, New Jersey

Florin Grigorian, MD (Question 29)
Assistant Professor of Ophthalmology
Case Western Reserve University
Rainbow Children's Hospital
Cleveland, Ohio

Paula Grigorian, MD (Question 24)
Pediatric Ophthalmologist
Center for Pediatric Ophthalmology and Adult
Strabismus
Rainbow Babies & Children's Hospital
University Hospitals Eye Institute
Assistant Professor of Ophthalmology
Case Western Reserve School of Medicine
Cleveland, Ohio

Suqin Guo, MD (Questions 8, 10, 15, 33, 42)
Associate Professor
Pediatric Ophthalmology
Clinic Director
Institute of Ophthalmology & Visual Science
Rutgers—New Jersey Medical School
Newark, New Jersey

Sheryl M. Handler, MD (Questions 6, 7)
Pediatric Ophthalmology
Encino, California

Denise Hug, MD (Question 11)
Associate Professor
University of Missouri Kansas City
Children's Mercy Hospital
Section of Ophthalmology
Kansas City, Missouri

William R. Katowitz, MD (Questions 47, 48)
Assistant Professor of Clinical Ophthalmology
The Perelman School of Medicine
The University of Pennsylvania
Philadelphia, Pennslyvania

Albert S. Khouri, MD (Question 45)
Assistant Professor of Ophthalmology
Program Director, Ophthalmology Residency
Associate Director, Glaucoma Division
Rutgers—New Jersey Medical School
Newark, New Jersey

Paul D. Langer, MD, FACS (Questions 16, 49)
Associate Professor of Ophthalmology
Institute of Ophthalmology and Visual Science
Rutgers—New Jersey Medical School
Newark, New Jersey

Steven J. Lichtenstein, MD, FAAP (Question 17)
Associate Clinical Professor of Surgery and
Pediatrics
University of Illinois College of Medicine at
Peoria & Chicago
Children's Hospital of Illinois
Illinois Eye Center
Immediate Past President, Peoria Medical
Society
Peoria, Illinois

Renelle Pointdujour Lim, MD (Question 44)
Assistant Clinical Instructor
SUNY Downstate Medical Center
Department of Ophthalmology
Brooklyn, New York

Robert W. Lingua, MD (Question 3)
Clinical Professor of Ophthalmology
Director, Pediatric Ophthalmology and
Strabismus
University of California, Irvine
Gavin Herbert Eye Institute
Irvine, California

William Madigan, MD, FACS (Question 4)
Vice Chief & Fellowship Director, Division of
Ophthalmology
Clinical Professor of Ophthalmology &
Pediatrics, George Washington University
Children's National Medical Center
Professor & Chief, Division of Ophthalmology
Uniformed Services University of the Health
Sciences
Washington, District of Columbia

María Ana Martínez-Castellanos, MD (Question 39)
Retina Department
Asociación Para Evitar la Ceguera en México
Hospital "Luis Sánchez Bulnes"
Universidad Nacional Autónoma de México
Mexico City, Mexico

Linda Nakanishi, MD (Question 41)
Assistant Professor
Pediatric & Family Ophthalmology & Strabismus
University of South Florida
Tampa, Florida

Leonard B. Nelson, MD, MBA (Question 26)
Wills Eye Institute
Department of Pediatric Ophthalmology and Ocular Genetics
Philadelphia, Pennsylvania

Nina Ni, MD (Questions 8, 10, 15, 33, 42)
Wills Eye Hospital
Thomas Jefferson University
Philadelphia, Pennsylvania

Christina M. Ohnsman, MD (Question 18)
Department of Ophthalmology
Reading Hospital
Wyomissing, Pennsylvania

Scott E. Olitsky, MD (Questions 24, 25, 28, 29)
Chief of Ophthalmology, Children's Mercy Hospital
Professor of Ophthalmology
University of Missouri—Kansas City School of Medicine
Kansas City, Missouri

Catherine A. Origlieri, MD (Question 45)
Pediatric Ophthalmology Fellow
Children's National Medical Center
George Washington University
Washington, District of Columbia

Nicole Pritz, MD (Question 23)
Ophthalmology Resident
The Institute of Ophthalmology and Visual Science
New Jersey Medical School
Newark, New Jersey

Luke Rebenitsch, MD (Question 28)
Cornea and Refractive Surgery Fellow
Durrie Vision/University of Kansas Medical School
Department of Ophthalmology
Kansas City, Kansas

Ronald Rescigno, MD (Question 13)
Assistant Professor of Ophthalmology
Institute of Ophthalmology and Visual Science
Rutgers—New Jersey Medical School
Newark, New Jersey

Dorothy J. Reynolds, MD (Question 21)
Assistant Professor of Ophthalmology, Stony Brook Medicine
Division Chief of Pediatric Ophthalmology, Stony Brook Children's
Department of Ophthalmology
University Hospital and Medical Center
State University of New York at Stony Brook
Stony Brook, New York

James Reynolds, MD (Question 38)
Professor and Chairman
University at Buffalo, Department of Ophthalmology
Ross Eye Institute
Buffalo, New York

Carol L. Shields, MD (Questions 34, 35, 36, 37)
Professor of Ophthalmology
Thomas Jefferson University
Co-Director of Ocular Oncology Service
Wills Eye Institute
Philadelphia, Pennsylvania

Roman Shinder, MD (Question 44)
Associate Professor of Clinical Ophthalmology
Director of Oculoplastics
SUNY Downstate Medical Center
Brooklyn, New York

Melissa A. Simon, MD (Question 1)
Pediatric Ophthalmology Fellow
Casey Eye Institute
Oregon Health and Sciences University
Portland, Oregon

Jonathan C. Song, MD (Question 19)
Assistant Professor of Ophthalmology
Division of Pediatric Ophthalmology & Adult Strabismus
Division of Cornea, Cataract & External Diseases
The Wilmer Eye Institute
The Johns Hopkins School of Medicine
Baltimore, Maryland

Roger E. Turbin, MD, FACS (Question 14)
Associate Professor
Rutgers—New Jersey Medical School
Institute of Ophthalmology and Visual Science
Newark, New Jersey

Rudolph S. Wagner, MD (Question 1, 22, 23, 40, 43)
Clinical Professor and Director of Pediatric Ophthalmology
Institute of Ophthalmology and Visual Science
Rutgers—New Jersey Medical School
Newark, New Jersey

Foreword

Pediatric ophthalmology has become a well-recognized and established subspecialty. Recent advances in the understanding of such areas as visual development in the preverbal child, ocular genetics, amblyopia and strabismus have resulted in increased knowledge and clarification of these subjects and, therefore, better care of the pediatric patient. Yet, for those involved in caring for the pediatric patient, attempting to analyze and evaluate all the clinical material presented in a variety of academic venues can be time consuming and overwhelming. These same individuals try to streamline the process of attaining the necessary information to assist them in patient care by asking questions of their colleagues, "the experts in their field." Dr. Rudolph Wagner, an outstanding pediatric ophthalmologist, one of those "experts," has done a superior job in editing the *Curbside Consultation in Pediatric Ophthalmology*. He has successfully assembled numerous colleagues in pediatric ophthalmology to ask questions and answer them in the everyday care of the pediatric patient. This edition of *Curbside Consultation* will appeal to residents-in-training, fellows, as well as seasoned pediatric ophthalmologists in the successful care of their patients.

Leonard B. Nelson, MD, MBA
Wills Eye Institute
Department of Pediatric Ophthalmology and Ocular Genetics
Philadelphia, Pennsylvania

Introduction

I continue to be amazed by the depth and diversity of knowledge required of those involved in pediatric health care. They need to know as much about dermatology as cardiology, as anxious caregivers await the diagnosis and treatment that will cure their children. It should not surprise anyone that pediatricians prescribe far more medications for the treatment of the various forms of pediatric conjunctivitis then do ophthalmologists. The need to know exists for eye care.

The purpose of this book is to augment the diagnostic and management skills of busy health-care providers for disorders of vision and pediatric ocular disease. An expert panel of ophthalmologists in all subspecialties, and others involved in the eye care of children was assembled to contribute chapters on relevant topics. Each chapter is unique, concise, and delivers practical information about preferred practice patterns based on current scientific information with the goal of improved outcomes for your patients.

The "49 Questions" answered in this book were selected by a panel of pediatricians for their relevance to everyday practice. Pertinent issues, from how to perform vision screening in the office to the management of eye trauma, including corneal abrasions and minor lid lacerations, are included. The chapters are succinct enough to provide a ready reference for formulating a plan for the treatment of a child present in the office.

The information to answer a concerned parent's questions about dyslexia, and how you might be able to test a child for it, is there for you. As are selected references, for those who care to delve into the topic in greater detail. Lists of available resources are included to aid in your management of numerous disorders.

I envision this book being utilized daily in a busy pediatric or primary care practice, clinic, or emergency department. Comprehensive ophthalmologists who see children in their practices will also find this book extremely useful. I hope the readers will enjoy reading this book as much as the authors, including myself, have enjoyed writing it.

SECTION I

VISION SCREENING

QUESTION

WHAT ARE THE NORMAL DEVELOPMENTAL MILESTONES FOR VISION IN INFANTS?

Rudolph S. Wagner, MD and Melissa A. Simon, MD

Briefly explained, normal development of vision occurs when an infant's eyes respond to visual stimuli and successfully communicate a stimulus to the brain. As we cover the various milestones for normal vision development in infants (Table 1-1), remember that all of these milestones are likely to be reached later in children who were born prematurely.

Visual development begins with response to light. Premature infants of 30 weeks, gestational age at birth will blink in response to light. A pupillary light reflex (pupillary constriction to light) can be noted even in premature babies as young as 31 weeks, gestational age. However, a newborn's pupils will be small and will respond poorly. Constriction in response to light can be difficult to see without magnification, and it is brief. Use bright light to elicit this reflex, preferably in a dimly lit room. Pupils that dilate rather than constrict with light have a paradoxical response that requires investigation by an ophthalmologist.

Parents often ask what their infants can see. Newborns have about 20/400 vision, which can be explained to parents as equivalent to seeing the big E on an eye chart. At birth, the area of the retina responsible for central vision does not yet have the photoreceptors needed for clearer vision. These photoreceptors redistribute over the first year of life to achieve approximately 20/20 vision by 1 year of age.

During the first month of life, a newborn is most responsive to a human face and light, seeing objects held about 30 cm in front of the face. To understand why objects must be at this distance to be in focus, it is important to know that most children are born hyperopic, or farsighted, and become increasingly hyperopic during the first 7 years of life. Farsightedness is a bit of a misnomer because images will be foggy at a distance as well as near. So how does the infant overcome this fog? A child's eye can correct a large amount of hyperopic refractive error without glasses by mechanisms of accommodation. Infants in the first month of life lack the ocular motor control

Wagner RS. *Curbside Consultation in Pediatric Ophthalmology: 49 Clinical Questions* (pp 3-6)
© 2014 SLACK Incorporated

Table 1-1
Normal Developmental Milestones

Age	Normal Developmental Milestones
Birth	• Blink in response to light (as early as 30 weeks, gestational age) • Poor but present pupillary light reflex (as early as 31 weeks, gestational age) • 20/400 vision • May exhibit transient vertical ocular misalignment and sunsetting, a tonic downward movement of both eyes
First month	• Responsive to a human face and light, seeing objects held about 30 cm in front of the face in best focus • Highly variable ocular alignment
6 weeks	• Start accommodating to see objects at a variety of distances • Fix-and-follow eye movements begin • Eye contact usually begins
3 to 4 months	• Ocular alignment is maintained
12 weeks	• More developed convergence allows exploration of distant and 3-dimensional objects
5 months	• Blink in response to threat
5 to 7 months	• Can distinguish a caretaker or familiar relative from others by sight
7 to 10 months	• Develop a finer focus and can see small objects and detailed facial features • Permanent eye color is usually established at month 9
1 year	• 20/20 vision

to accommodate a continuous range to see objects at various distances. Their accommodation is tonic. This means that most objects at most distances will be foggy until the infant is a little older.

A 6-week-old infant can start accommodating to see objects at a variety of distances. Although some newborns can fix and follow with horizontal tracking. This ability is more clearly recognizable by the sixth week of life if a bright target or light is used. Infants of 6 weeks can usually track vertically and circularly as well. The infant becomes more interested in patterns and will watch mobiles, although a human face is still the best object for stimulating an infant to fixate. The parent's or primary caregiver's face is the best of all. Normally, fix-and-follow movements are not smooth in young infants. If a child cannot fix and follow by 3 or 4 months, particularly during periods of heightened attention, the child should be evaluated by an ophthalmologist.

Eye contact normally begins at 6 weeks of age, although up to 8 weeks is still normal. An infant older than 8 weeks who responds to a parent's voice but does not make eye contact should be referred to an ophthalmologist.

By 12 weeks of age, accommodation and convergence are more fully developed, and infants begin to focus on their hands, which helps them learn hand-eye coordination and recognize distances as they start to grab at objects they can see. These skills help the infant build an understanding of 3-dimensional space and orientation.

By 5 months of age, an infant should blink in response to threat, although this response will likely be difficult to notice on examination. Blinking responses to both light and threat are learned responses. Around 5 to 7 months of age, an infant can distinguish a caretaker or familiar relative from others by sight.

Between 7 and 10 months of age, infants develop a finer focus and can see small objects and detailed facial features. Depth perception is more advanced. At 1 year of age, most children have 20/20 vision, though they can't communicate that on a vision screening.

Parents frequently ask about eye movements and crossed or lazy eyes, wondering what is normal. Explain that both eyes must be aligned and work together for depth perception, which is called *binocular stereopsis*. Alignment during the first month of life is highly variable, with intermittent deviations occurring frequently. Sometimes the eyes will turn in (esotropia) or turn out (exotropia). Healthy newborns may also exhibit transient vertical ocular misalignment and sunsetting, a tonic downward movement of both eyes. This should not be confused with the true setting-sun sign of hydrocephalus. In the setting-sun sign, both ocular globes are deviated downward, the upper lids are retracted, and the white sclera may be visible above the iris. In the first year of life, exotropias are the more common type of strabismus, or misalignment. A persistent variable exotropia occurs frequently in children with developmental delay. After the first year of life, esotropias become more common. Most infants, however, are able to maintain ocular alignment by 3 to 6 months, and some ophthalmologists feel that an infant should not have any misalignment by 4 months of age. However, if you or a parent notices misalignment at 3 months or a head turn when a child looks at an object straight ahead, the child should be referred to an ophthalmologist. Ocular pathology or a cranial nerve palsy could cause such a strabismus. Strabismus also may occur when one eye lacks good vision.

Nystagmus—rhythmic pendular or jerk movements of the eyeballs—is never a normal finding, although it is sometimes a benign condition. Nystagmus can be first noticed in infants 2 to 3 months of age. These eye movements are not present at birth and usually suggest that both eyes have poor vision (unlike strabismus). Roving or wandering eye movements are a particularly bad sign that require immediate work-up with an ophthalmologist.

Dissociated nystagmus—in which one eye has a greater amplitude or frequency—may be a sign of a chiasmal glioma or of a condition termed *spasmus nutans*. Spasmus nutans is a benign condition consisting of nystagmus, head nodding, and torticollis. The nystagmus in spasmus nutans is usually described as shimmering (small amplitude and high frequency), but it can also be asymmetrical and variable depending on head position. Onset for spasmus nutans is usually within the first 2 years of life, and it usually spontaneously resolves by age 3 or 4 years. Although it is a benign condition, chiasmal or suprachiasmal tumors can cause a similar presentation.

Nystagmus can be confused with *opsoclonus*, which is a flutterlike, random eye movement that may be normal in neonates. Rarely, opsoclonus can be a sign of neuroblastoma. The rapid and unpredictable eye movements noted in opsoclonus are believed to be caused by a paraneoplastic process in neuroblastoma, which can also cause myoclonus and ataxia.

Another sign of poor visual development is the oculodigital reflex, which is forceful or constant eye rubbing, an attempt by the infant to stimulate the nerves in the back of the eye to fire manually because they are not responding to light. In addition to intrinsic problems with the eye or brain, deprivation of visual stimuli can lead to poor visual development, such as in the case of a cataract or a ptotic lid that prevents light from getting to the retina in the back of the eye.

Parents frequently ask about their child's eye color and if it will change over time. Iris coloration in most newborns is a shade of gray. This will usually darken over time to blue or brown. Around 9 months of age, the permanent eye color is usually established. *Heterochromia*, or a difference of color between the 2 eyes, may indicate a pathologic condition. For example, infants with congenital Horner's syndrome may have a lighter colored iris on the side with eyelid ptosis and a miotic pupil.

When you examine a nonverbal child's eyes, check the external eyes for ptosis, proptosis, or masses. Look at pupils for reactivity or anisocoria (asymmetry), and confirm a normal red reflex. To evaluate motility and estimate visual acuity, examine both eyes together and separately. If a child cries or loses the ability to fix and follow when one eye is covered, that reaction suggests pathology in the uncovered eye. Use toys with bright colors, flashing lights, patterns, or high contrast to capture an infant's visual attention. Because the photoreceptors are developing, infants prefer to view items with large contrast differences, such as toys with large black and white stripes or brightly colored toys.

Suggested Readings

American Academy of Ophthalmology. Pediatric Ophthalmology and Strabismus: Basic and Clinical Science Course. Singapore: *American Academy of Ophthalmology.* 2009:45-46, 165-166, 451-456.

Hyvärinen L, Jacob N. Infants with normal visual development. *Dr. Lea and Children's Vision.* Jan 9, 2011. http://drlea-hyvarinen.com/2011/01/09/infants-with-normal-visual-development. Accessed April 21, 2012.

Nelson LB, Rubin SE, Wagner RS, Breton ME. Developmental aspects in the assessment of visual function in young children. *Pediatrics.* 1984;73:375-381.

WHAT IS PEDIATRIC OFFICE PHOTOSCREENING? WHEN SHOULD I USE IT?

Robert W. Arnold, MD, FAAP

Children still go blind from amblyopia, even in advanced pediatric practices in America, but the future looks bright.

Amblyopia is characterized by deficient brain learning of visual acuity as a result of imperfect image formation during the first decade of life. The primary causes are constant strabismus (usually esotropia), blocked images (ie, by pediatric cataract), and by defocused images as a result of high farsightedness, high astigmatism, severe nearsightedness, and particularly unequal refractive error (anisometropia). Two-thirds of amblyopia cases are associated with excess refractive error. Almost all cases of strabismic amblyopia have an amount of ocular misalignment that is obvious to parents.

Photoscreening is a technique for analyzing the images of reflected light through the pupils to determine refractive error, media clarity, and ocular alignment. It evolved from the Bruckner test and retinoscopy; therefore, photoscreening detects the potential causes of amblyopia, not necessarily the acuity defect that results in a reduction in monocular or bilateral visual acuity. Photoscreening specifically finds the treatable components of amblyopia. Photoscreening can reliably be done in children as young as 9 months.

Photoscreening can outperform routine acuity screening in the pediatric office.[1] In busy pediatric practices near Vanderbilt University, conventional acuity vision screening referred a similar percent of preschool children as did the MTI Polaroid photoscreener placed alternately in the practice environment. The predictive value from photoscreening was 75%, whereas the predictive value from acuity screening in that series was zero. Once demographic data are entered, or uploaded into a photoscreener, the actual screening can take less than 5 seconds, whereas careful, patched, monocular critical line acuity screening takes 3 minutes to perform in a preschooler, and threshold acuity screening can take 5 minutes or more.

Wagner RS. *Curbside Consultation in Pediatric Ophthalmology: 49 Clinical Questions* (pp 7-9) © 2014 SLACK Incorporated

Figure 2-1. 2012 commercially available photoscreeners. From left to right, iScreen, SPOT, and PlusoptixS09. The iScreen has keyboard name, age, and clinic input; uses a triangulation focusing light similar to the MTI Polaroid photoscreener; quickly exposes 2 images; and allows ethernet upload for prompt, centralized-reading-center interpretation. SPOT by Pediavision has keyboard entry of ID number, first and last names, sex, and birthdate with screen view alignment and focus. SPOT provides software interpretation and WiFi or USB flash download of reports and uploads of grouped patients or screening-program interpretation criteria. Plusoptix is widely validated and is the most recent Linux-based version from prior Windows/Firewire versions (the S04 and S08). Aiming the Plusoptix off the accompanying computer screen and user-modifiable referral criteria by age are used to generate practice-customized printout reports for parents. Widespread validation of iScreen and SPOT are pending.

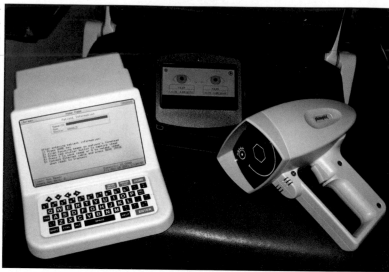

The prevalence of amblyopia to a degree of 20/40 visual acuity or worse in one or both eyes is about 2% to 3% of an American community. The prevalence of amblyopia risk factors is about 6 times that. Good photoscreening programs have been able to achieve a referral rate of 5% to 7%, with a positive predictive value of 75% to 95% in preschool children.[2]

Commercially available photoscreeners have either instant computer interpretation or prompt expert reading center analysis online. Reports can be generated and charted and/or given to parents to assist with obtaining a reliable confirmatory examination for referred patients. Examples of commercially available photoscreeners in 2012 are the PlusoptiX (Plusoptix Inc), iScreen (iScreen Vision, Inc), and the SPOT (PediaVision) (Figure 2-1). Remote autorefractors are the Suresight Vision Screener (Welch Allyn) and the Retinomax (S4OPTIK).

Jack Bellows, the founder of the iScreen photoscreener invested to produce the photoscreening CPT code (99174-) with an RVU of 0.69 to allow pediatric practices to bill for photoscreening services. Photoscreeners are available for purchase or for lease with per-screening interpretation fees.

Early photoscreening (age 1 to 2 years) may have the potential to reduce amblyopia severity even more than detection of amblyopia in preschool screening in children aged 3 to 5 years.[3] Treatment success is better for children detected between ages 3 to 5 years compared with those detected between ages 5 to 6 years.

The current commercially available photoscreeners can fit well in the workflow of a pediatric office. Nurses can become proficient at using the devices on cooperative children with a short learning curve. More experienced screeners can get valid results from infants, toddlers, and even developmentally delayed and autistic patients.[4] The actual screening times can be less than 5 seconds after demographic input or upload.

Photoscreening is an early part of the American Academy of Pediatrics (AAP)-recommended series of age-appropriate screening measures.[5] It follows newborn red reflex and infant fixation observation and must be followed by careful, patched-monocular acuity screening after age 5 to 6 years into school.

The Alaska Blind Child Discovery has been validating state-wide photoscreening since 1996 and recommends that each child get photoscreened between ages 12 to 24 months and again between ages 3 and 4 years.[6] Photoscreening is a valid and faster alternative to monocular acuity screening for kindergarten entry. Photoscreening should be attempted on older children with developmental delays such that they cannot yet perform a reliable monocular visual acuity.

With widespread, early photoscreening as a part of AAP guideline screening, amblyopia vision impairment should be eliminated.

The time for pediatric office photoscreening is now.

References

1. Salcido AA, Bradley J, Donahue SP. Predictive value of photoscreening and traditional screening of preschool children. *J Aapos*. 2005;9(2):114-120.
2. Longmuir SQ, Pfeifer W, Leon A, Olson RJ, Short L, Scott WE. Nine-year results of a volunteer lay network photoscreening program of 147 809 children using a photoscreener in iowa. *Ophthalmology*. 2010;117(10):1869-1875.
3. Kirk VG, Clausen MM, Armitage MD, Arnold RW. Preverbal photoscreening for amblyogenic factors and outcomes in amblyopia treatment: early objective screening and visual acuities. *Arch Ophthalmol*. 2008;125(4):489-492.
4. Arnold RW, Armitage MD. Performance of four new photoscreeners on pediatric patients with high risk amblyopia. *JPOS*. 2014;51(1):46-52.
5. Miller JM, Lessin HR. AAP: instrument-based pediatric vision screening policy statement. *Pediatrics*. 2012;130(5):983-986.
6. Arnold RW. Alaska Blind Child Discovery. www.ABCD-Vision.org. Accessed January 23, 2014.

Suggested Readings

BPEDS, Friedman DS, Repka MX, et al. Prevalence of amblyopia and strabismus in white and african american children aged 6 through 71 months the baltimore pediatric eye disease study. *Ophthalmology*. 2009;116(11):2128- 2134. e2121-e2122.

MEPEDS. Prevalence of amblyopia and strabismus in african american and hispanic children ages 6 to 72 months the multi ethnic pediatric eye disease study. *Ophthalmology*. 2008;115(7):1229-1236. e1221.

Repka MX, Kraker RT, Beck RW, et al. A randomized trial of atropine vs patching for treatment of moderate amblyopia: follow-up at age 10 years. *Arch Ophthalmol*. 2008;126(8):1039-1044.

Swanson J. Eye examination in infants, children and young adults by pediatricians: AAP policy statement. *Ophthalmology*. 2003;110(4):860-865.

Swanson J, Committee on Practice and Ambulatory Medicine. Use of photoscreening for children's vision screening (AAP Policy Statement). *Pediatrics*. 2002;109(3):524-525.

QUESTION

3

WHAT ARE THE BEST METHODS TO SCREEN FOR STRABISMUS IN THE PEDIATRICIAN'S OFFICE?

Robert W. Lingua, MD

Why Screen for Strabismus?

A child with an ocular misalignment (strabismus) will avoid the appreciation of diplopia by suppression. *Suppression* means that there is an active inhibition of visual transmission to the visual cortex from one eye when binocular viewing is interrupted by ocular misalignment. When eyes are misaligned, different objects are perceived by each eye pointing in a different direction. To avoid this confusion, the cortical projection of one is suppressed. This results in, at best, alternate suppression (when the child easily alternates use of the 2 eyes, fixating with one and suppressing the other) and, at worst, amblyopia (occurs when one eye is consistently suppressed, such that upon monocular viewing with that eye, vision is poor, or, as commonly labeled, lazy). The neuropharmacology of this event is not well understood. The success of treating amblyopia due to strabismus rapidly declines after 5 years of age. Early diagnosis of an ocular misalignment is therefore paramount.

Screening visual performance in a child should include an assessment of alignment, range of movement, and of each eye's ability to see independently. This chapter will address the assessment of eye alignment and range of movement; the assessment of acuity, including photoscreening for the detection of amblyopia risk factors, is addressed in a separate chapter.

It is common in pediatric ophthalmology to discuss screening techniques according to the relative maturity of various age groups. I will not do that here because I believe it is most useful to the pediatrician to have a few universal methods that are consistently reliable for infant to toddler. We will assume that older children will cooperate with commands given to assess alignment, ocular rotations, and binocularity.

Library Resource Center
Renton Technical College
3000 N.E. 4ᵗʰ Street
Renton, WA 96056

Wagner RS. *Curbside Consultation in Pediatric Ophthalmology: 49 Clinical Questions* (pp 11-16)
© 2014 SLACK Incorporated

Figure 3-1. Spinning lights in a globe.

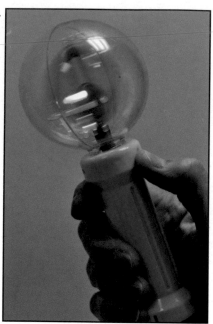

The suggested order of examination will progress from the least threatening, remote assessment, to a closer interaction. A thorough screening will require only 1 to 2 minutes. The 5 key maneuvers are listed next. The attention-getting device you use is *essential*. If you use an unattractive object, or worse, an obnoxiously bright pen light, poor cooperation will follow, parents will lack confidence in your findings, and you will become frustrated. Invest in a globe with spinning lights, available in large department stores or online for about $5 (Figure 3-1). It is infallible in securing the attention of any child, making the process more enjoyable for all. Also, have your cell phone handy, with the camera mode set to flash. You can use it to play the latest cartoon as a fixation device, or to capture a photo of the corneal light reflex. Presenting a picture to the parent will prove invaluable when discussing your diagnosis. Although modern binocular photoscreening devices are programmed to assess alignment, in my assessment, the false positive rate is high. The following clinical maneuvers are more accurate.

The 5 key maneuvers, in order of performance, are as follows:

1. Corneal light reflex

2. Ocular rotations

3. Bruckner test

4. Cover test

5. Stereopsis test

Corneal Light Reflex

The most common method to screen for ocular alignment has been the subjective assessment of the symmetry of the corneal light reflex relative to the dark pupil. Commonly, a parent will present with a strong belief that a child's eyes are crossing, and you'll need a rapid, objective way to address his or her fears.

The corneal light reflex test, if done with a quick flash of the penlight, often is insufficient to allay the parent's concerns. A bright light is not at all interesting to children, and it's perfectly understandable that their first response will be to look away from it. This is a difficult situation when you are trying to assess the light reflex or show the parent that you know what you are doing. Further, small deviations can be missed with this test. As little as a 1-mm asymmetry in the light reflex is equivalent to 10 degrees of misalignment, or about 20 prism diopters. But suppression and amblyopia can occur with as little as 4 to 8 prism diopters or about a 0.25-mm offset! This cannot be detected by gross observation of the corneal light reflex alone. The corneal light reflex test is only going to pick up large deviations, whereas clinically significant smaller ones may be undetectable. This test should be used in addition to the tests that follow, but not as the sole test of ocular alignment.

Rather than trying to describe to the parent what you are seeing, a better option is to use your cell phone camera to capture an image for discussion. Typically, these phones are familiar to the child. Often children will enter the exam room playing with the parent's cell phone. A flash photo at a distance of 2 feet will yield remarkable images for your interpretation. When epicanthal folds suggest esotropia to the untrained eye, a reproducible demonstration to the parent that there is centration of the light reflex in the pupils can assure him or her that if the eyes are turning (as they think), it's not there constantly. You can show him or her how to monitor the child at home in this manner. Of course, there may be a strabismus that the parent doesn't appreciate, and it is of equal value in that case. You can also download the images from your camera to the electronic medical record for future reference, or to justify a referral. If you are successful with the spinning globe and phone, continue with that approach to the documentation of ocular rotations. You can steady the child's chin with your thumb and take photos in any other gaze position.

Ocular Rotations

It is equally important to capture a photo in right and left gaze, using the spinning light globe to secure the child's attention. Forms of strabismus exist where the eyes are straight in primary position but deviated in other positions of gaze (eg, Duane's syndrome and fourth cranial nerve palsy) (Figure 3-2). Therefore, don't be too reassuring until you get a photo of right and left gaze. Take care to present only one stimulus at a time. Voicing a noisy stimulus in one direction and then holding a fixation target in another quickly confuses the child.

If the child is under 1 year of age, the status of ocular rotations can be quickly assessed by generating rotations or an optokinetic nystagmoid movement with either of the following 2 methods.

DOLL'S EYES

While holding the child with a hand under each armpit and each thumb steadying the chin, the child is turned right, left, up, and down while the examiner uses his or her face and sounds to attract his or her attention. Observe the symmetry of ocular rotation into these 4 fields of gaze created as the child maintains fixation on your face. Noisy targets (you) are helpful when the goal is to stimulate ocular rotations, but not to assess acuity.

ROOM-BASED OPTOKINETIC NYSTAGNUS

To elicit an optokinetic nystagmus (OKN), support the child under the arms as described previously, steady the chin with your thumbs, and rotate yourself along with the child. Observe the child's eye movement as he or she views the fixed objects in the room over your shoulder (Figure 3-3). Observe the ocular rotation as the child fixes on an object and follows it (slow pursuit movement), then refixates (fast saccadic movement) on the next target. This maneuver is valuable

Figure 3-2. (A) Misalignment (vertical) seen in side gaze (B) could be missed on straight-ahead gaze.

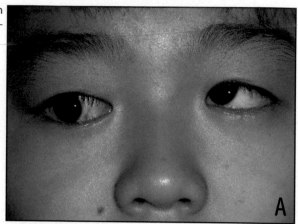

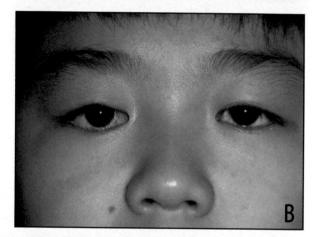

Figure 3-3. Support the child under the arms and rotate, observing the eye movements as he or she gazes at objects over your shoulder.

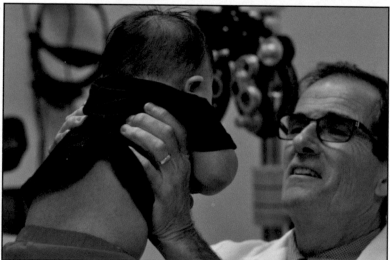

in the 4- to 6-month-old with poor fixation reflexes and delayed visual maturation (DVM), as opposed to poor acuity. A child with true vision loss will not be able to demonstrate this reflex, and a child who appears to have vision loss as deduced by visual inattention can be proven to be sighted if he or she can demonstrate this room-based OKN.

Bruckner Test

Best performed after dilation but adequately done in a dimly lit room, this test offers an assessment of the relative intensity of the red light reflex, reflecting off the fundus and through the pupil, when viewed through the direct ophthalmoscope. Look at the pupillary red reflex from both eyes simultaneously from a distance of approximately 3 feet through your direct ophthalmoscope set to 0. Holding the spinning globe near his or her face will keep attention during your observation. Assess the relative size, color, and brightness of the 2 reflexes. Any significant asymmetry warrants referral.

The American Academy of Pediatrics publishes this testing method as part of a "See Red" campaign and the site can be accessed at http://aappolicy.aappublications.org/cgi/content/full/pediatrics;122/6/1401.

Another consumer web site is www.knowtheglow.org, which encourages parents to examine the red reflex seen in most family photos.

Cover Test

The gold standard for the diagnosis of a constant ocular misalignment is the cover test. Again, the key to success is the use of an interesting target. An eye is covered and any shift in ocular position by the uncovered eye to find the target you present is a positive test. Get the interest of the child, then cover the right while observing the left, and then switch hands and cover the left while you observe the right. You may want to use different targets for each eye due to the child's attention span. Stickers of cartoon characters on a pencil are inexpensive and can be readily interchanged. The success of the test is not only dependent on the ability of the target to maintain attention during the test, but also on the quality of the cover used. Typically, a child will not tolerate a black paddle-type eye occluder, and using your thumb as the cover while the hand steadies the forehead may be more successful (Figure 3-4). The cover can't be so interesting as to distract attention from the target. This test screens for alignment at near fixation, the most important position for visual development. Because strabismus may exist only on distance fixation (eg, intermittent exotropia), diagnosis of these conditions may have to await their ability to cooperate with fixation on distant projected targets while the cover test is performed. The cover test simultaneously screens for possible amblyopia, suspected when the child consistently objects to covering one eye and demonstrates a strong preference for viewing with only one eye on multiple trials. Equal objection to cover is not diagnostic of amblyopia, but rather of a symmetric preference for seeing with either eye in the absence of amblyopia.

Stereopsis Test

In order for a child to appreciate 3D vision, or stereopsis, both eyes have to be aligned to permit simultaneous perception. Stereopsis testing has been frequently used in the screening of preschool children for strabismus. It is of value only when positive because false negative responses are

Figure 3-4. Steady the head and use your thumb as an occluder.

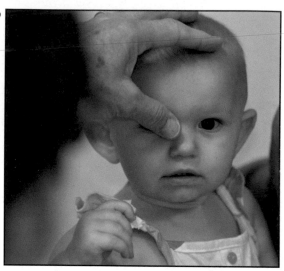

common. Although most infants and toddlers will not permit the polarizing tinted glasses to be placed on their face, the test can be attempted with the glasses reversed. When there is a startle response or an attempt to grasp the test object in the book (fly, butterfly, or smiley face), you can conclude that (a) gross stereopsis (depth perception) is intact, (b) an acceptable alignment exists for binocularity at least on near fixation, and (c) a deep amblyopia is not present.

Suggested Reading

Committee on Practice and Ambulatory Medicine Section on Ophthalmology, American Association of Certified Orthoptists, American Association for Pediatric Ophthalmology and Strabismus, American Academy of Ophthalmology. Eye examination in infants, children, and young adults by pediatricians. *Ophthalmology.* 2003;110(4):860-865.

How Do I Make a Diagnosis of Amblyopia?

William Madigan, MD, FACS

Amblyopia is not just poor vision in the conventional sense. Amblyopia is poor vision resulting from lack of development of appropriate synapses and cells in the visual cortex due to inadequate stimulation during infancy and childhood. David Hubel and Torsten Wiesel were awarded the Nobel Prize in 1981 for their work in cats and monkeys, which first identified the relationship between optimal visual stimulation and cortical neuronal cell and network development. The earlier in childhood the visual development is handicapped, the more profound the effect on development in the visual cortex. Conversely, the earlier the intervention to correct amblyopia, the faster and more complete the response to therapy. After 9 years of age, the visual cortical maturation has historically been considered complete and not subject to manipulation either for better or worse vision. In recent years, there is new research using penalization therapy together with oral dopamine to determine whether later interventions may still reduce amblyopia. This study should clarify if therapy for amblyopia in patients older than 9 years of age is worthwhile.

Any condition that interferes with stimulation of the central vision (served by the macula and fovea) may lead to amblyopia. Peripheral vision, on the other hand, is not susceptible to amblyopia. Prior to 3 months of age, the binocular fusion system in the midbrain has not developed sufficiently to hold the 2 eyes in parallel alignment, and a variety of strabismus conditions may be observed, all of which disappear after 3 months of age unless there is a more serious underlying condition. Children under 9 years, when presented with the diplopia resulting from misaligned eyes, suppress the image in the deviated eye, and that eye becomes amblyopic.

Some common problems that lead to the development of amblyopia are listed in Table 4-1.

Alignment

When you first enter the room, look to see if the child is alert and interested in his or her surroundings. Examine the reflection of the overhead lights on the corneas and look for a symmetric

Wagner RS. *Curbside Consultation in Pediatric Ophthalmology: 49 Clinical Questions* (pp 17-20)
© 2014 SLACK Incorporated

Table 4-1
Common Causes of Amblyopia

Strabismus (misalignment of the eyes)*
Anisometropia (large differences in refractive error between the 2 eyes)
Isoametropia (large refractive differences that are the same in both eyes)
Visual pathway disturbance (corneal scar, cataract, vitreous opacity)*
Monofixation syndrome (diagnosis of exclusion)

Any office assessment for amblyopia should include the following:
- Evaluation of eye alignment
- Pupillary and anterior segment (cornea, lens) examination
- Examination of the quality of the red reflex
- Best evaluation of vision possible for the age of the patient

*These conditions result in the deepest amblyopia with the most profound negative effect on visual development.

pupillary light reflex slightly displaced nasally in each pupil an equivalent amount (positive angle kappa—the difference between the anatomic and visual axis of the eye) (Hirschberg method of evaluation of alignment). Shining a penlight held in front of your face toward the child will also provide the best reflex. Sometimes a red filter can be held in front of the penlight to reduce the child's discomfort and promote better fixation on the light by the child. Clucking or cooing sounds may also lead the preverbal child to pay better attention to your fixation light. This is best done as the first part of the eye exam, before anything else is done that may interfere with the child's binocular fusion system responsible for maintaining eye alignment. Any asymmetry of the reflex may indicate strabismus. Alignment can be further evaluated by presenting a series of small objects of interest to the child while alternately covering one eye, then the other. If a shift of the immediately uncovered eye is observed, this is evidence of strabismus. The typical rule is "1 toy, 1 look," so you will need a box full of small toys. Any detectable strabismus may be assumed to be causing amblyopia to develop in the less favored eye.

Pupil and Anterior Segment Examination

Sometimes a profound blockage of light along the visual axis may result in a mild afferent pupil defect (APD) (reverse Marcus-Gunn) on pupil exam, but a large APD usually only manifests as a result of a chronic retinal detachment or, more likely, a severe problem with the optic nerve such as optic nerve hypoplasia (ONH). These should not be confused with amblyopia, although dense amblyopia itself may result in a subtle APD.

Any abnormal physical findings determined by examination that interfere with the passage of focused light to the macula and fovea may be presumed to cause amblyopia in patients during the amblyogenic period under 9 years of age. Light may be blocked by something like a cataract or corneal scar. The light may arrive at the retina too blurry to provide proper stimulation due to optical refractive error. Amblyopia may occur in one or both eyes.

Red Reflex

The clarity of the visual axis and any severe refractive errors can be assessed through evaluation of the red reflex at any age. The direct ophthalmoscope is set at a neutral diopter reading based on the examiner's refractive error, and the reflex from the patient's pupil is observed from approximately 18 inches away. Asymmetry in the reflex's appearance between eyes, lack of a bright orange-red reflex, or a dull reflex should result in referral for ophthalmic evaluation. Automated photoscreeners rely on this reflex to identify abnormalities requiring further investigation. The cause of the lack of a normal red reflex can often be determined by direct examination of the anterior eye. A corneal opacity over the pupil that blocks the view of the iris and lens will clearly be amblyogenic. A cloudy lens forming a cataract can be identified just behind the iris plane. Problems in the vitreous and retina may result in an abnormal red reflex but require dilation and better optical devices available to ophthalmologists to diagnose.

Vision Assessment

In neonates, typically we record blinks to light, or BTL, because often even normal newborns have poor tracking ability and visual acuity in the 20/200 to 400 range. In older preverbal infants, we must rely on their observed fixation behavior. From 1 to 3 months of age, we observe if the child fixes and follows an interesting visual object (recorded as F&F) with each eye separately. This is an approximate visual evaluation. Fixation behavior can appear equally good when compared between the 2 eyes, and yet they may differ in vision substantially (20/40 in one eye and 20/200 in the other when alternate research methods—impractical in clinical practice—such as preferential looking are used to more accurately determine vision).

After 3 months of age, when the binocular system and fusional control are developing well, we can compare the fixation preference between eyes. We conduct a cover/uncover fixation assessment. If the eyes are straight, we must evaluate the child's behavior while each eye is covered in turn. If the child vigorously objects and tries to avoid the cover of 1 eye compared with the other, or loses interest and doesn't follow the object well when the presumptively better eye is covered, we may indirectly assume there is an inequality between the eyes. This may represent amblyopia. Sometimes this eye preference is obvious (Figures 4-1 and 4-2), but it may be more subtle and require repetitive testing to determine a pattern.

If any strabismus is present, the cover/uncover test can easily detect a fixation preference. While the nonfixated eye is covered, we simultaneously evaluate if the covered eye drifts away while we also present an object of interest to the child to fixate with the uncovered eye. We continue to assess the observed/uncovered eye as we uncover the fellow eye. Does the child maintain fixation with the observed eye, or does he or she immediately switch fixation to the newly uncovered eye and not maintain fixation with the observed eye? If fixation is central, steady (no nystagmus or inattentive wandering due to poor sight) and maintained (no fixation switching with uncover), we report this as CSM. Children lose interest quickly, so remember the "1 toy, 1 look" rule. This test should be done simultaneously with the alignment assessment.

For children older than 2 to 3 years of age, you may use the tumbling E or Allen picture method to evaluate monocular vision. Some children are shy and initially may be better at pointing to the picture you ask them to identify on a near vision card rather than looking at a distance and reporting what they observe. Isolate the line size you wish to test and ask the child to point to the bird or ask, "where is the picture of a car?" You can provide the family a handout to practice with at home between visits.

Figure 4-1. Covering the preferred eye for vision.

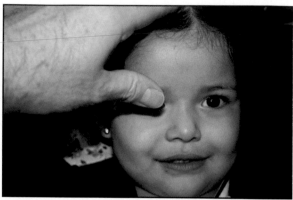

Figure 4-2. Covering the amblyopic eye.

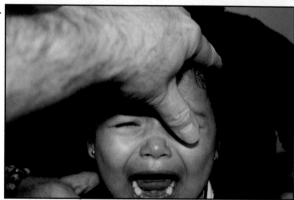

Older children (usually over 4 to 5 years of age) may be tested in the standard manner with Snellen acuity charts at distance and/or near. Additionally, the Titmus stereotest requires all systems to be working perfectly to achieve a maximum score. All 9 circles being correctly selected as 3D (40 sec of arc) is only possible if both eyes are perfectly aligned and have 20/20 vision independently.

Asymmetric vision should be considered to result from amblyopia until a complete assessment can be performed by an ophthalmologist.

Suggested Readings

Basic and Clinical Science Course. *Section 6: Pediatr Ophthalmol Strabismus. Part V and VI.* San Francisco, CA: American Academy of Ophthalmology; 2003-2004.

Preferred Practice Patterns Committee, Pediatric Ophthalmology Panel. *Amblyopia.* San Francisco, CA: American Academy of Ophthalmology; 1997.

Von Noorden GK. Amblyopia: multidisciplinary approach. Proctor Lecture. *Invest Ophthalmol Vis Sci.* 1985;26:1704-1716.

QUESTION

5

WHAT ARE THE ESSENTIALS OF THE EYE EXAMINATION THAT
SHOULD BE INCLUDED IN ROUTINE PEDIATRIC OFFICE VISITS
FOR SPECIFIC AGE GROUPS?

Dawn Duss, MD

Diagnosing pediatric subspecialty problems can be challenging and, at times, overwhelming. Pediatric ophthalmology is not generally emphasized in residency, but children with vision problems are encountered frequently in clinical practice. Improper or delayed diagnosis can result in permanent visual damage, and it is critical that pediatricians feel confident in their ability to screen for the most visually important conditions of childhood. In each age group, certain elements of the clinical examination should be emphasized.

Birth to Age 1 Month: The Red Reflex

When examining the red reflex using a direct ophthalmoscope, lower the room lights and be sure to stand far enough away from the patient to illuminate both eyes simultaneously. Attend to both quality and symmetry. Is the reflex dull or bright? Is it the same in each eye? Are there opacities present on retroillumination? Any lens opacity greater than 2 mm in size is visually significant, and even opacities smaller than 2 millimeters may become so, especially if centrally located in the visual axis. Visually significant congenital cataracts must be removed within the first 1 to 2 months of life so timely diagnosis and referral to a pediatric ophthalmologist is crucial (Figure 5-1).

A white reflex, or leukocoria, is equally as concerning as a dull one. The differential diagnosis of leukocoria includes conditions such as cataract, retinoblastoma, optic nerve or chorioretinal coloboma, persistent hyperplastic primary vitreous, and retinal detachment, all of which should be referred to a specialist in an expedited manner. Photoleukocoria, or a white pupil reflected in photographs (Figure 5-2), should prompt full evaluation, even if leukocoria is not witnessed in

Wagner RS. *Curbside Consultation in Pediatric
Ophthalmology: 49 Clinical Questions* (pp 21-27)
© 2014 SLACK Incorporated

Figure 5-1. Bilateral congenital cataract diagnosed within 1 week of life.

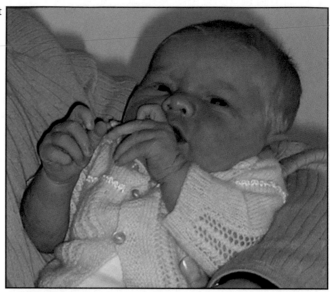

Figure 5-2. (A) Photoleukocoria noticed by mother. (B) Group B retinoblastoma in the right eye. *(continued)*

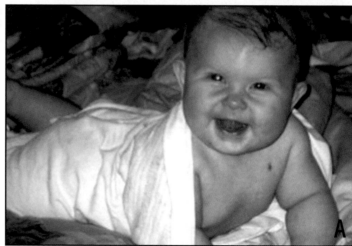

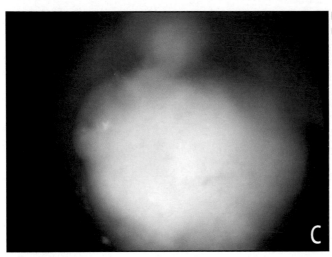

Figure 5-2 (continued). (C) Group D retinoblastoma in the left eye.

the pediatrician's office. Parental descriptions of leukocoria at home are remarkably accurate and should be taken seriously. 56% of retinoblastoma patients present with a white reflex.

Age 2 to 6 Months: Central, Steady, and Maintained Visual Behavior

Newborn babies will rarely attend to visual stimuli consistently, but by 2 to 3 months of age, fixation ability should develop to approximately a 20/600 to 20/300 Snellen acuity level. By 3 to 4 months, accommodation and focused attention should be maintained, and babies should attend to toys within their central visual field. When testing fixation, it is important to observe both monocular and binocular visual behavior. Monocular fixation should be assessed for quality and accuracy (is fixation steady or is nystagmus present?), location (central versus eccentric), and duration (maintained versus sporadic). In a child with poor vision in one eye only, occlusion of the better seeing eye will often result in an angry reaction in the child. The child may cry and push away your occluder because you have taken away his or her only seeing eye. Binocular fixation preference compares the vision of one eye with the other and can identify amblyopia in potential conditions such as anisometropia, ptosis, or strabismus.

Ocular deviations are common in infancy, with nearly 70% of newborns showing intermittent exodeviation in the first few weeks of life. However, deviations that do not resolve by 3 months of life warrant further investigation, before sensory adaptations develop. In the immature visual system, ocular misalignment will result in suppression and permanent disruption of binocularity.

Age 6 to 12 Months: Buphthalmos

Primary infantile glaucoma occurs in 1 of every 10,000 live births, with the onset of symptoms before age 1 year in 86%. Most cases are sporadic, with a higher incidence in males, but a family history of glaucoma increases risk of disease. It is believed to evolve from primary trabeculodysgenesis resulting in abnormal outflow of fluid from the eye. The clinical manifestations of infantile glaucoma are determined largely by the age of onset and the degree of intraocular pressure elevation. Corneal enlargement and/or clouding, photophobia, epiphora, and

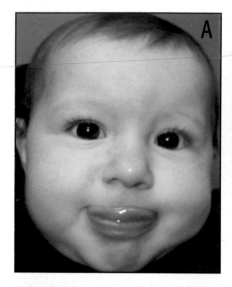

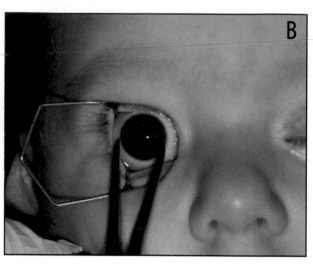

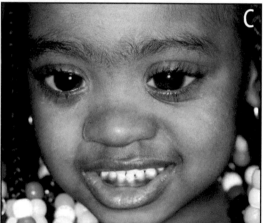

Figure 5-3. (A) Subtle bilateral buphthalmos. (B) Corneal diameter 12.50 x 12.25 millimeters. (C) Dramatic bilateral buphthalmos associated with severe glaucoma (delayed diagnosis).

blepharospasm are the most characteristic findings. The epiphora present in congenital glaucoma is associated with corneal clouding and light sensitivity, whereas epiphora in congenital dacryostenosis is more often associated with copious mucous production and matting of eyelashes. Enlargement of the cornea can be subtle, especially in bilateral cases, and can go unnoticed, even by family members (Figures 5-3A and 5-3B). Even severe buphthalmos may be gradual in nature. Families may mistake this appearance for benign primary megalocornea and fail to alert a physician (Figure 5-3C). Unilateral cases tend to present earlier, because asymmetric corneal enlargement is more obvious. Careful inspection of the cornea in the office, even with a penlight, will reveal linear or circumferential breaks in Descemet's membrane, called *Haab's striae,* as well as areas of clouding, consistent with corneal edema. Corneal clouding may be dramatic when pressure rises rapidly over a short period of time but essentially absent if pressure changes are gradual. It may even be present at birth if pressure elevation occurs in utero.

Secondary glaucoma results from an underlying primary condition such as anterior segment dysgenesis (aniridia, Peters' anomaly, Axenfeld-Reiger syndrome), infectious/inflammatory disease, chromosomal anomaly, or systemic disorder. All children with phacomatoses (Sturge-Weber syndrome, neurofibromatosis, von Hippel-Lindau disease), metabolic disease (Lowe syndrome, mucopolysaccharidoses, cystinosis), and connective tissue abnormalities (Marfan syndrome, Weill-Marchesani syndrome, Ehlers-Danlos syndrome, osteogenesis imperfecta, sulfite oxidase deficiency) should be evaluated for signs of elevated intraocular pressure. Children with Rubinstein-Taybi syndrome, Pierre Robin syndrome, and congenital Toxoplasmosis, Other, Rubella, Cytomegalovirus, and Herpes simplex virus (TORCH) infections are also at risk.

Age 3 to 5 Years: Amblyopia

Derived from the Greek *amblys* "dull" and *ops* "eye," amblyopia refers to poor vision caused by abnormal visual development secondary to improper visual stimulus. The most common forms of amblyopia are deprivation, strabismic, and anisometropic. *Deprivation amblyopia* occurs most often in the setting of intraocular abnormalities or severe ptosis, whereas *strabismic amblyopia* arises from ocular misalignment. *Anisometropic amblyopia* results when there is a substantial difference in refractive error between the eyes, promoting visual development in one eye at the expense of the eye with the blurred visual image. Children with anisometropic amblyopia often have straight eyes and function well in school and play. There are few, if any, outward signs or symptoms. Thus, anisometropic amblyopia often presents at an older age, when patients are more refractory to treatment. Early diagnosis and treatment remains a challenge. The key to timely intervention lies in accurate visual acuity testing. Clinical pearls include the following:

- Complete occlusion of the opposite eye for monocular testing. Be sure to use an opaque patch or tape. Covering one eye with your hand is not adequate! Children who cannot see will cheat. A child who objects to monocular testing has amblyopia until proven otherwise.

- Use matching symbols. Many preschool-aged children are shy, especially in their doctor's office. Allowing them to match pictures by pointing instead of talking puts the child at ease and eliminates the fear of conversing with the doctor. Making it a matching game instead of a test improves attention and interest in the task, promoting adequate cooperation even in some 2 year olds.

- Never test with single optotypes (only one symbol or letter at a time). Linear acuity (several symbols or letters at a time) is preferable to single optotype testing because single optotype presentation overestimates level of acuity. This is especially true in children with amblyopia, who tend to perform 1 to 2 Snellen lines better when presented with single optotypes as compared with linear. This has been called the *crowding phenomenon* and has been linked to the large receptive field associated with amblyopia.

Age 5 to 10 Years: Intermittent/Incomitant Strabismus

Most clinicians feel confident in their ability to detect large-angle, constant misalignment, but intermittent strabismus can be just as damaging to the development of binocularity. By definition, intermittent strabismus is not manifest at all times and may not be readily apparent unless fusion is disrupted. Control may vary depending on fatigue or the distance at which alignment is tested. Thus, cover-uncover testing should be performed on all children and should be performed for both distance and near viewing targets (Figure 5-4). Likewise, some forms of strabismus, including restrictive and paretic, are apparent only in nonprimary positions. Always look for incomitance, or increased misalignment, in different positions of gaze. An acute esotropia that increases in side

Figure 5-4. (A) Orthophoric for near viewing target. (B) Intermittent exotropia when
viewing at a distance.

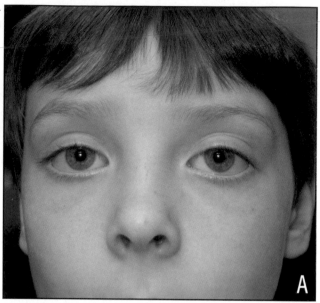

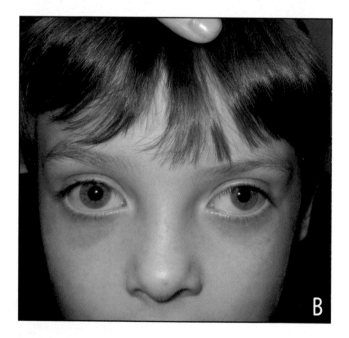

gaze suggests a CN VI paresis and should raise concern for the possibility of intracranial pathology. Even well-controlled intermittent deviations and phorias should be referred for further evaluation. Small latent deviations (phorias) may decompensate into large manifest deviations, and it is
important to intervene before suppression develops. For intermittent exotropes, an increase in the
size of the exodeviation indicates progression and should prompt escalating therapy. Patients with
larger preoperative deviations have a poorer outcome, so intervention is best when misalignment
is small.

Suggested Readings

Gezer A, Nasri N, Gozum N. Factors influencing the outcome of strabismus surgery in patients with exotropia. *J AAPOS*. 2004:8(1):56-60.

Papadopoulos M, Khaw PT. Childhood glaucoma. In: Taylor D, Hoyt CS, eds. *Pediatric Ophthalmology and Strabismus*. 3rd ed. Philadelphia, PA: Elsevier Saunders; 2005:458-471.

Reynolds JD, Olitsky SE. Pediatric glaucoma. In: Wright KW, Spiegel PH. *Pediatric Ophthalmology and Strabismus*. 2nd ed. New York, NY: Springer-Verlag; 2003:483-498.

Stout AU. Pediatric eye exam. In: Wright KW, Spiegel PH. *Pediatric Ophthalmology and Strabismus*. 2nd ed. New York, NY: Springer-Verlag; 2003:57-67.

WHAT IS DYSLEXIA, AND HOW IS IT TREATED?

Sheryl M. Handler, MD

Nearly 40% of students initially experience difficulties in learning how to read. Parents may be the first ones to realize that their child is struggling with learning to read. At that time, parents may ask you to evaluate their child to provide information and referrals for further evaluation and treatment. This chapter is designed to provide you with information and strategies to help parents of children with dyslexia.

Children may show difficulties in early reading for many reasons, including deficits in oral language, lack of background knowledge, inadequate instruction, insufficient reading practice, or a true reading disability.

Reading disability is the most common learning disability. A learning disability is a lifelong condition affecting the way the brain processes information. Reading disability can also be called *dyslexia* and the medical term is *reading disorder*. Dyslexia is not a transient developmental lag, but a lifelong condition.

Dyslexia is a learning disability that effects language. Children with dyslexia have difficulties with multiple language skills, including difficulties with written word decoding and recognition, reading fluency, and pronouncing words. They often have secondary problems with comprehension, spelling, and writing. Because children with dyslexia tend to read less, they often have reduced growth in their vocabulary and background knowledge.

Dyslexia is frequently an unexpected reading difficulty in an otherwise bright child. Dyslexia is common. It is estimated that as many as 1 out of every 5 people or 20% of children in the United States have some degree of dyslexia. It occurs in boys and girls nearly equally, but boys are diagnosed significantly more often than girls, possibly because they act out more often.

Dyslexia is hereditary. Approximately 40% of siblings, children, or parents of an affected individual will have dyslexia. If one family member has dyslexia, early language development and

Wagner RS. *Curbside Consultation in Pediatric
Ophthalmology: 49 Clinical Questions* (pp 29-34)
© 2014 SLACK Incorporated

school performance should be carefully followed in all younger family members. The educational progress of children who show risk factors for dyslexia, such as prematurity, neurological problems, language, or any developmental delay, should also be carefully monitored.

Dyslexia often coexists with other learning disabilities, most commonly *dysgraphia* (writing disability) and sometimes with motor skill and coordination difficulties called *dyspraxia*. Students with dyslexia frequently encounter difficulties with math word problems and learning a foreign language.

Problems with attention, concentration, executive function, and verbal working memory often greatly exacerbate dyslexia. Twenty to 40% of people with dyslexia have attention deficit disorder/ attention deficit hyperactivity disorder (ADD/ADHD) and vice versa. Children with dyslexia often become frustrated and their self-esteem may plummet. These children may feels less capable than they actually are, become discouraged about continuing school, and may develop anxiety or depression. If any of these problems are suspected, early evaluation and management are recommended.

Children with dyslexia are often bright, analytic, and creative; have an ability to think outside the box; and may be gifted in other areas. Because of their disability, they often learn to persevere.

Historically, dyslexia was thought by some to be a vision-based disorder, and some people continue to believe this. However, 50 years of scientific evidence has shown that eye and visual problems do not cause or increase the severity of dyslexia and children with dyslexia do not have more visual problems than children without dyslexia. Over this time, research has repeatedly demonstrated that dyslexia is a language-based learning disorder.

There is strong evidence that most people with dyslexia have a problem distinguishing and separating the sounds in spoken words (phonological deficit). Recent functional magnetic resonance imaging (fMRI) scans have shown that children with dyslexia use different areas of the brain compared with typical readers. Using this pathway makes it difficult to understand the connection between the sounds and the letters of the alphabet, and secondarily to use the alphabet to decode the written word. Also, some children with dyslexia have trouble rapidly naming objects, whereas other children have both a phonological deficit and difficulty with rapid naming, creating a double deficit.

Many educators have not received sufficient training in dyslexia and so do not recognize that it is a language-based disorder rather than a vision-based disorder. This incorrect classification has been propagated frequently by promoters of vision-based treatments. Educators often look for letter and word reversals to identify dyslexia instead of looking for difficulties with language, learning the letters and their sounds, sounding out words, and spelling. This can lead to delays in recognition and treatment, and frustrations for the parents.

Parents and teachers should look for signs of possible dyslexia listed in Table 6-1.

Until recently, most elementary education teacher preparation college programs have had minimal instruction on the speech sound system, language structure, reading development, reading problems, early signs of possible dyslexia, and methods of teaching students with dyslexia. Fortunately, the International Dyslexia Association (IDA) is committed to improving teacher training. The IDA understands that learning to teach reading, language and writing requires changes in the current teacher curriculum to provide this comprehensive education. In 2010, the IDA developed standards for colleges and universities to guide preparation, certification, and professional development of teachers who teach reading. Many programs are rising to this challenge and are now becoming certified. Better prepared and informed educators will improve the outcomes for all students, including those with dyslexia.

Table 6-1
Signs of Possible Dyslexia

- Language delays
- Difficulties with rhymes
- Difficulty learning the names and sounds of the letters
- Difficulty sounding out words
- Difficulty with sight word recognition
- Not learning to read as expected
- Slow reading

- Trouble with comprehension
- Trouble with spelling
- Avoidance of reading, especially out loud
- Frustration with schoolwork and homework
- Problems with attention

Pediatrician's Role

Parents may become concerned when they notice that their child is struggling to remember letters, and words or how to read, spell, or do their homework. Parents may experience additional frustration because schools often don't identify the problem early or provide extra help to improve it. At that time, parents may turn to you. You can serve a number of important functions for children with dyslexia and their families.

You can assess the whole child at the well-child examination. You can determine whether there is a history of prematurity or birth problems and/or, a family history of speech and language problems or dyslexia, and you can assess for medical problems that could affect a child's ability to learn or may have caused school absences. Early developmental screenings in your office may identify early language or learning concerns. The evaluation should include vision and hearing screening and evaluation for ADD/ADHD, autism spectrum disorder, anxiety, depression, or other problems.

You should refer your patient to a pediatric ophthalmologist for a thorough evaluation if anyone suspects a possible vision problem or if your patient fails vision screening. This will ensure that there are no eye or vision disorders, because some of these children may have a visual problem that masquerades as a learning problem, or they may have a treatable visual problem along with their primary learning problem. This is one of the reasons that a pediatric ophthalmologist should be a part of the evaluation team.

Visual problems occur in approximately 5% to 10% of early elementary students and 25% of high school students. Treatable ocular conditions include strabismus, amblyopia, convergence or focusing deficiencies, and refractive errors. A need for glasses may make it difficult to see the board or to read. Many of these conditions can be treated with glasses and generally will show benefit very quickly.

Medications or counseling can be used to improve attention problems and other conditions such as anxiety or depression. Enhanced attention may contribute to improvement in the child's reading and overall performance in school.

You should encourage parents to trust their instincts, learn about reading problems, become their child's advocate, and take steps to seek an educational evaluation from a school or an outside specialist as soon as possible.

If you are familiar with the local school districts, federal and state laws, and the rights of students with dyslexia and other specific learning disabilities, you can help to advocate for the child.

By writing a letter to the school, you may be able to assist the family in requesting an evaluation. A formal evaluation is needed to determine the diagnosis and determine a treatment plan. A psychoeducational school evaluation is performed to gain a better understanding of the child's strengths and weaknesses, and the severity of the problem, to recommend specific interventions, and to determine whether the child has a learning disability that is severe enough to be eligible for special education and support programs. The evaluation will provide a road map on which evidence-based interventions and accommodations are based.

If the student has other medical or neurological conditions or has not been making progress after prior psychoeducational evaluation, diagnosis, and interventions, you might want to request that the child obtain an evaluation by a behavioral pediatrician or neuropsychologist. These examinations provide a broader assessment of brain function, than does a school psychoeducational evaluation, to identify the underlying causes of the disorder.

After a diagnosis has been made, you can facilitate obtaining further medical and psychological evaluations and treatments as necessary. Many myths and misconceptions surround dyslexia and its treatment, and it is important for you to provide information and dispel these myths. (For additional information on this topic, see Question 7.) You may want to give the parents a resource list including informational Web sites, books (included at the end of this section), and compile a personalized list of local specialists.

Treatment of Dyslexia

Children who are identified early can be treated early, and early intervention is often successful. Students whose dyslexia is identified and addressed in kindergarten or first grade have an approximately 90% chance of improving to grade level. It is important to identify and begin to treat children before they leave third grade to have the best chance at academic success, but it's never too late.

Children with dyslexia require lessons by a highly skilled teacher in small groups of 2 to 5 students at the same level. Programs should include individualized, highly structured, intensive daily instruction and practice. These programs should continue long enough to have a positive effect that will endure. Children with dyslexia need language explained in patterns that are logical, explicit, systematic, sequential, and multisensory. Explicit instruction means that children are not expected to infer keys skills or knowledge. Multisensory learning involves the use of visual, auditory, kinesthetic and tactile pathways simultaneously to enhance memory and learning of written language. Information on multi sensory programs can be found at the International Dyslexia Association (www.interdys.org), the Alliance for Accreditation and Certification of Structured Language Education, Inc (www.allianceaccreditation.org), the International Multisensory Structured Language Education Council (www.imslec.org), and the Academy of Orton-Gillingham Practitioners and Educators (www.ortonacademy.org).

These programs should include explicit training in the 5 reading skills of: phonemic awareness, phonics, fluency, vocabulary, comprehension, plus writing and spelling. The brain learns best by practice. Practice in oral reading, not silent reading, improves reading fluency. Unfortunately, struggling readers tend to avoid practice, but they actually need to practice much more.

Children with dyslexia also require accommodations in school. Accommodations allow access to higher-level thinking and reasoning skills. Some of these include: a computer or other technology, recorded books, text-reading software, note-takers, spell-checkers, extended time for test taking, a special quiet room for testing, testing alternatives, and preferential seating.

An outside educational therapist or experienced, specially trained reading tutor may be helpful for some children who require additional help outside of school.

Sometimes we forget to look at the whole child and only look at his or her weaknesses. Parents should identify their child's social, athletic, and academic strengths and concentrate on activities in which their child excels. With early identification and treatment, children with dyslexia can experience high achievement in life. Working together, children, parents, and members of the medical and educational communities can formulate and oversee a prescription for success.

Suggested Readings

Handler, SM. *A Parent's Guide to Dyslexia (Reading Disability).* Available at: http://www.aapos.org/resources/learning_disabilities.

Handler SM, Fierson WM, Section on Ophthalmology; Council on Children with Disabilities; American Academy of Ophthalmology; American Association for Pediatric Ophthalmology and Strabismus; American Association of Certified Orthoptists. Learning Disabilities, Dyslexia, and Vision Technical Report. *Pediatrics.* 2011;127(3):e818-e856. http://pediatrics.aappublications.org/content/127/3/e818.full.pdf+html.

Shaywitz SE, Shaywitz BA. The science of reading and dyslexia. *JAAPOS.* 2003;7(3):158-166.

Informational Books

Levine M. *A Mind at a Time.* New York, NY: Simon and Schuster; 2002.

Schonfeld A, Niendam T, Schiltz K. *Beyond the Label: A Guide to Unlocking a Child's Educational Potential.* New York, NY: Oxford University Press; 2012.

Shaywitz S. *Overcoming Dyslexia: A New and Complete Science-Based Program for Overcoming Reading Problems at Any Level.* New York, NY: Knopf; 2003.

Silver L. *The Misunderstood Child: Understanding and Coping with Your Child's L.D.* (4th Ed) New York, NY: Three Rivers Press; 2006.

E-Book

Dyslexia Toolkit - National Center for Learning Disabilities. Available at: http://www.ncld.org/images/content/files/Dyslexia_101_E-Book.pdf.

Movie on Dyslexia

The Big Picture: Rethinking Dyslexia. Information is available at: http://thebigpicturemovie.com/.

Informational Web Sites

All Kinds of Minds by Mel Levine, MD
www.allkindsofminds.org

American Academy of Ophthalmology
www.aao.org

American Academy of Pediatrics
www.aap.org

American Assoc. of Pediatric Ophthalmology &
  Strabismus
www.aapos.org

American College Testing—Students With Disabilities
www.actstudent.org/regist/disab

American Speech-Language and Hearing Association
www.asha.org

Association of Educational Therapists
www.aetonline.org

Bookshare
www.bookshare.org

College Board Services—Students With Disabilities
www.collegeboard.com/ssd

Educational Records Bureau
www.erblearn.org

Educational Testing Service - Students With Disabilities
www.ets.org/disabilities

International Dyslexia Association
www.interdys.org

Learning Ally
www.rfbd.org

Learning Disabilities On Line
www.ldonline.org

Lindamood-Bell
www.lindamoodbell.com

National Center for Learning Disabilities
www.ncld.org

Orton-Gillingham
www.orton-gillingham.com

Quackwatch
www.quackwatch.com

Reading Rockets
www.readingrockets.org

Schwab Learning
www.greatschools.org

University of Michigan—Dyslexia Help
www.dyslexiahelp.umich.edu

US Department of Education
www.ed.gov

Yale Center for Dyslexia & Creativity
www.dyslexia.yale.edu

QUESTION

7

DOES VISION THERAPY OR COLORED LENSES BENEFIT DYSLEXIA?

Sheryl M. Handler, MD

Pediatricians are often asked to evaluate children who are experiencing difficulties learning to read. Because dyslexia and other learning disabilities are chronic conditions with no simple cure, they have spawned a wide variety of scientifically unsupported diagnostic and treatment procedures. When parents are anxious to find solutions, friends, teachers, other health providers, or the media may suggest expensive and unproven treatments such as vision therapy or colored lenses. Parents may ask you to comment on these methods although you may not know a lot about them. This chapter is designed to provide you with information you can use to assure parents that vision therapy and colored lenses do not benefit children with dyslexia.

Historically, dyslexia was thought by some to be a vision-based disorder, and some people continue to believe this. When a teacher notices that a student has problems with writing or fluent oral reading, the teacher may believe that the child has an eye-tracking problem. Actually, children with dyslexia often lose their place while reading because they struggle to decode a letter or word combination, lack comprehension, or have difficulties with memory and attention, not because of an eye-tracking problem.

Many teachers still look for letter and word reversals to identify dyslexia. It is a common misconception that children with dyslexia see letters upside-down or backwards. People with dyslexia do not see things backwards. They actually view text the same way you and I do.

Research has demonstrated that letter and word reversals and skipping words and lines are symptoms, not causes, of reading disorders. They have been shown to result from language deficiencies rather than visual disorders.

Wagner RS. *Curbside Consultation in Pediatric Ophthalmology: 49 Clinical Questions* (pp 35-39)
© 2014 SLACK Incorporated

Vision Therapy

Behavioral optometrists, who advocate vision therapy for learning disabilities and dyslexia, claim that more than 60% of problem learners have undiagnosed vision problems contributing to their difficulties. The current optometric policy statement on the topic of learning disabilities asserts that "...vision therapy does not directly treat learning disabilities or dyslexia." Despite the lack of evidence, it continues "...vision therapy is a treatment to improve visual efficiency and visual processing, thereby allowing the person to be more responsive to educational instruction." Regrettably, the subtleties of the wording of this statement are lost to the public.

In disagreement with the optometric viewpoint, a large number of studies have indicated that subtle eye or visual problems are not critical factors in dyslexia. In fact, 50 years of scientific evidence has concluded that eye and visual problems do not cause or increase the severity of dyslexia. Vision problems can interfere with the process of reading, but children with dyslexia have the same visual function and ocular health as children without such conditions.

Behavioral optometrists use techniques they call vision therapy, which they define as an attempt to develop or improve visual skills and abilities; improve visual comfort, ease, and efficiency; and change processing of visual information. An optometric vision therapy program is described as consisting of supervised in-office and at-home reinforcing exercises performed over weeks to months and may include training glasses (ie, very low-power reading glasses). Behavioral optometrists believe that training glasses and vision therapy will make reading more efficient. They also believe that every child would benefit from training glasses, and they recommend that training glasses be used preventatively to avert the stress of near work. In addition to eye exercises and training glasses, behavioral optometrists also use prisms, filters, patches, electronic targets, specialized instruments, balance boards, metronomes, and computer programs in vision therapy.

Pediatric ophthalmologists and orthoptists do use glasses, patching, filters, and atropine in the evidence-based treatment of amblyopia and strabismus. However, ophthalmologists and orthoptists do not use these techniques as a treatment for dyslexia, because there is no evidence that these modalities are effective for this diagnosis. Because visual problems do not underlie dyslexia, approaches designed to improve visual function by training are misdirected.

A pediatric ophthalmologist should be a member of the dyslexia evaluation team. Sometimes a child may also have a treatable visual problem accompanying or contributing to their primary reading or learning dysfunction. It is important for pediatric ophthalmologists to evaluate for near vision problems, including high hyperopia, convergence insufficiency, or focusing difficulties as these problems can occasionally masquerade as dyslexia. Missing these problems could cause long-term consequences from assigning these patients to incorrect treatment categories. Treatable ocular conditions include strabismus, amblyopia, convergence and/or focusing deficiencies, and refractive errors.

Convergence insufficiency is a condition characterized by a patient's inability to maintain proper binocular eye alignment as an object approaches from distance to near. It is often an asymptomatic condition, but rarely children develop eyestrain, headache, blurred vision, double vision, or moving vision with prolonged near work. Some children with symptomatic convergence insufficiency may only read for short periods of time before they develop discomfort and become reluctant to read. Some children may close or cover one eye when they are reading to try to relieve this eye strain. This behavior may cause teachers or parents to think that the child may have ADD/ADHD or dyslexia. However, it is important to understand that even if a child is diagnosed with symptomatic convergence insufficiency, that may cause reluctance to read, it does not cause dyslexia. There are children with both convergence insufficiency and dyslexia. In those children, treating the convergence problems may relieve the eye strain but does not treat the underlying reading disorder.

Convergence exercises or vision training has been demonstrated to be beneficial for symptomatic convergence insufficiency. Most of the treated children will improve in a few weeks. It is important to understand that convergence exercises may make reading more comfortable and allow longer periods of reading, but it is not a treatment for dyslexia.

If a child is found to have symptomatic convergence insufficiency, most pediatric ophthalmologists recommend at-home convergence exercises, including computer convergence eye exercises with periodic follow-up office visits. If he or she continues to show signs and symptoms of convergence insufficiency after the in-home therapy or had difficulties with in-home treatment then in-office treatment should be considered. On the other hand, most behavioral optometrists recommend the more expensive and time consuming in-office convergence training with at-home reinforcement as their first treatment.

In-office vision therapy has been shown to have a large placebo effect. For example, the placebo vision therapy group in the Convergence Insufficiency Treatment Trial showed a 35% positive response rate. Thus, it could be expected that over a third of your patients who participate in vision therapy for any reason would have this positive placebo effect and could provide positive anecdotes to you or their friends.

The optometric literature has been thoroughly reviewed multiple times over the years, including several exhaustive reviews by optometrists. These reviews have revealed that vision therapy is not evidence-based with the exception of convergence insufficiency. There is no valid evidence that training glasses or vision therapy prevents the development of visual disorders, allows children to be more responsive to educational instruction, or is an effective primary or adjuvant treatment for dyslexia or other learning disabilities. On the topic of dyslexia, the purported benefits of vision therapy often can be explained by the placebo effect, increased time and attention, maturation changes, or the educational remedial techniques with which they usually are combined. In spite of these facts, behavioral optometrists have heavily promoted vision therapy directly to the public through the media. Behavioral optometrists often rely on testimonials and anecdotal evidence to convince parents that vision therapy is effective, and they often overstate the therapy's effectiveness and the types of problems it may address.

Despite the lack of corroborating research findings with statistical validity, vision therapy is popular and pervasive. Unfortunately, using ineffective methods of treatment may give parents and teachers a false sense of security that a child's reading difficulties are being addressed. These evaluations and therapy sessions are extremely expensive. They waste family or school resources and time and may delay or reduce the amount of time available for appropriate instruction.

Colored Lenses and Filters

At a national meeting in 1983, Irlen proposed treatment with tinted (colored) lenses for a specific group of adults with reading problems suffering from what she originally called the "scotopic sensitivity syndrome," now also called "Irlen syndrome" or "Meares-Irlen syndrome." This is not a recognized medical syndrome. There are no clearly established criteria for making the diagnosis, and the only defining characteristic is the reported benefit of the colored filters themselves.

Supporters of Irlen syndrome contend that the syndrome affects 12% to 15% of the general population and 45% of those with learning problems. Perceptual dysfunctions are thought to cause light sensitivity and visual distortion interfering with attention, fluency, and comprehension. Irlen supporters believe that the colored lenses and filters reduce the offending wavelengths of light. Whereas, there has not been research to directly evaluate these statistics or hypotheses. Even Irlen supporters state that tinted lenses treat only perceptual symptoms or the visual component of reading problems and will not impact the phonologic deficits underlying most cases of reading disabilities.

In addition to improving reading, Irlen International Newsletters have credited their tinted lenses with helping individuals suffering from light sensitivity, discomfort, and distortions associated with a wide variety of neurologic, psychiatric, and ophthalmic conditions.

Studies have shown that the color selection of the lenses has shown poor test-retest consistency and that the tint selected needed to be changed in up to 25% of subjects within 1 year. Different tinted lens promoters use different methods of color selection. The Irlen method selects the lens or filter color by student preference, the Wilkins method uses the precision tint method, and Harris assesses each eye separately to determine the color of his ChromaGen lenses. There are apparently 16 different color ChromaGen lenses, although they all appear gray. The ChromaGen lenses were originally used to try to improve color deficiency and color blindness without true success, and they are now being promoted for the treatment of dyslexia.

The scientific studies that proponents of tinted lenses use as proof have shown serious methodologic flaws and are often scientifically invalid. Published studies do not support the use of tinted lenses and filters as a direct or indirect treatment for reading difficulties. Specifically, there is no valid evidence that Irlen, Wilkins, or ChromaGen lenses are helpful in the treatment of dyslexia. In fact, there are many studies demonstrating the lack of benefit. Colored lenses and filters may be ineffective, except that they act as a placebo. In spite of the lack of valid supporting evidence, these expensive methods are promoted to teachers and directly to the public.

Many children who have worn colored glasses have been teased or bullied, which may only further damage a child's self-confidence. Using expensive tinted lenses may give parents and teachers a false sense of security that a child's reading difficulties are being addressed and may delay proper evaluation and treatments.

Conclusion

The use of vision therapy and tinted lenses for dyslexia, clearly contradicts all of the research evidence that demonstrates that reading skills depend on language-based processes, such as phonological awareness.

No scientific evidence supports the use of training glasses, eye exercises, behavioral/perceptual vision therapy, or colored lenses and filters to improve the long-term educational performance in children with dyslexia.

Controversial therapies are frequently featured by the media. Aggressive promotion may convince parents to try these treatments. As advocates for your patients, you should inform parents that the scientific evidence shows that vision therapy and colored lenses do not benefit children with dyslexia. You should discourage parents from having their children participate in such unproven programs, saving valuable time and resources to be used for evidence-based educational therapies.

You should refer children with reading difficulties early in the evaluation process to a pediatric ophthalmologist to determine whether there are any eye or visual problems that may be contributing to their learning problems. The pediatric ophthalmologist on the dyslexia management team can also provide information to your patients and families that dyslexia is a language processing problem, not a vision problem, and that struggling readers need educational evaluation and remediation, not vision-oriented remedies such as eye exercises or colored lenses. Pediatric ophthalmologists can also help guide families of struggling readers to resources that are available in the community, in print, and on-line.

Referral for vision therapy or colored lenses is not supported by research. If your patient has undergone an evaluation and vision therapy or colored lenses have been recommended, you should advise your patient to be examined in second opinion by a pediatric ophthalmologist.

Suggested Readings

Barrett B. A critical evaluation of the evidence supporting the practice of behavioural vision therapy. *Ophthalmic Physiol Opt.* 2009;29:4-25.

Convergence Insufficiency Treatment Trial Study Group. Randomized clinical trial of treatments for symptomatic convergence insufficiency in children. *Arch Ophthalmol.* 2008;126(10):1336-1349.

Fletcher JM, Currie D. Vision efficiency interventions and reading disability. *Perspectives on Language and Literacy.* 2011;37(1):21-24.

Handler SM. *A Parent's Guide to Dyslexia.* Available at: http://www.aapos.org/resources/learning_disabilities_/.

Handler SM, Fierson WM, Section on Ophthalmology; Council on Children with Disabilities; American Academy of Ophthalmology; American Association for Pediatric Ophthalmology and Strabismus; American Association of Certified Orthoptists. Learning Disabilities, Dyslexia, and Vision Technical Report. *Pediatrics.* 2011;127(3):e818-e856. http://aappolicy.aappublications.org/cgi/reprint/pediatrics;127/3/e818.pdf.

Jennings AJ. Behavioural optometry: a critical review. *Optometry in Practice.* 2000;1(2):67-78.

Ritchie SJ, Della Sala S, McIntosh RD. Irlen colored overlays do not alleviate reading difficulties. *Pediatrics.* 2011;128(4):e932-e938.

SECTION II

CATARACTS

IF A CHILD HAS DEPRIVATION AMBLYOPIA, IS THERE ANYTHING THAT CAN BE DONE TO CORRECT IT? WHAT ARE THE CAUSES, SIGNS, AND SYMPTOMS?

Suqin Guo, MD and Nina Ni, MD

Amblyopia, also known as "lazy eye," refers to a decrease in vision in one or both eyes that does not improve when the refractive error is corrected (ie, with glasses). It is typified by a "crowding phenomenon," wherein the child is able to recognize individual letters better than a whole line on an eye chart. Amblyopia occurs in 2% to 4% of children. It is not associated with any significant organic or structural ocular anomaly, except in cases of deprivation amblyopia. Several types of amblyopia have been characterized according to the underlying cause(s).

Strabismus amblyopia occurs when either eye is not well aligned. Strabismus can result in, or be caused by, amblyopia. *Anisometropic amblyopia* occurs when there is a significant refractive error difference between eyes. *Deprivation amblyopia* is the least common form of amblyopia. It is, however, the most severe and difficult to manage. Deprivation amblyopia results from an obstruction or opacity in the visual axis, resulting in a blurry image. Opacities may be caused by congenital cataract, corneal edema, corneal scarring, congenital glaucoma, and ocular diseases of the retina and optic nerve. The most common causes of deprivation amblyopia are congenital cataract and corneal opacities. Loss of vision from deprivation amblyopia is more severe if visual input is obstructed by a cataract in one eye rather than both eyes.

What Are the Signs? How Should I Work It Up?

The most important clinical sign of amblyopia is decreased visual acuity (ie, blurry vision). A complete and thorough ocular examination should be done for children with blurry vision and a history of eye patching or eye surgeries (strabismus, cataract, or glaucoma). Relative afferent pupillary defect (Marcus Gunn pupil) occurs only rarely, even in severe amblyopia. Pupils should

Wagner RS. *Curbside Consultation in Pediatric
Ophthalmology: 49 Clinical Questions* (pp 43-46)
© 2014 SLACK Incorporated

Figure 8-1. A congenital cataract showing white opacity of the lens.

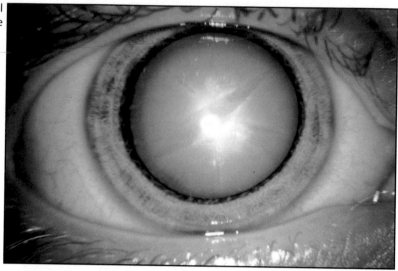

be checked for optic nerve disorders. A slit-lamp examination should be performed to check for the cornea edema or scarring, and any type of lens opacity (cataract) (Figure 8-1). The intraocular pressure (IOP) should be measured, as should the corneal diameter. One also needs to perform refraction and examine the optic nerve for glaucoma by checking the fundus for optic nerve and retinal pathologies. Ocular motility should be evaluated for strabismus. Retinoscopy is required to determine the need for spectacles.

Leukocoria, defined as a white pupil reflex, can be one of the most common presenting signs of congenital cataract (Figure 8-2). Haider et al[1] reported that 60% of children who presented with leukocoria had congenital cataracts (18% unilateral and 42% bilateral), 18% had retinoblastoma, and 4.2% had retinal detachment. Other causes included persistent hyperplastic primary vitreous (4.2%) and Coats disease (4.2%). Shields et al[2] reported that leukocoria can be a common presenting finding of retinoblastoma. It has been emphasized that leukocoria in children requires immediate attention and workups because a significant number will have a disorder that either threatens life or causes severe visual disability. Deprivation amblyopia can be associated with all of the above causes of leukocoria. If opacity of the ocular media prevents an accurate eye examination—including fundus—then B-scan ultrasound is warranted to rule out life-threatening intraocular tumors (ie, retinoblastoma).

Congenital cataracts can be associated with metabolic disorders, infections, and genetic disorders. Of bilateral congenital cataracts, one-third are inherited, and autosomal dominant is the most frequent mode of inheritance. It is also important to keep in mind systemic diseases associated with ophthalmologic pathology. The most common causes are hypoglycemia, infectious diseases (eg, Toxoplasmosis, Rubella, Cytomegalovirus, and Herpes Simplex—the TORCH infections), and trisomy syndromes (eg, Down and Edward syndromes). Therefore, children with congenital cataracts, especially those with bilateral involvement, require full metabolic, infectious, and genetic workups.

How Is Amblyopia Treated?

Occlusion (patching) of the eye with better visual acuity is the principal treatment for all forms of amblyopia. Another treatment is spectacle correction of significant refractive error or

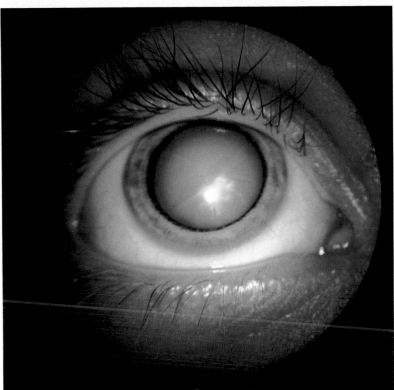

Figure 8-2. Leukocoria (white pupil reflex) is the most common presenting sign of congenital cataract.

anisometropia. For severe amblyopia, full-time (1 week for each year of age) patching is used; for moderate-to-mild amblyopia, part-time (2 to 6 hours/day until 9 to 11 years of age) patching is recommended. For children and parents who are not fully compliant with occlusion therapy, application of atropine (1%) into the better-seeing eye to blur vision can be used to improve vision in the amblyopic eye. This forces the brain to use the worse-seeing eye. Atropine can be as effective as patching therapy for mild-to-moderate amblyopia. For strabismus amblyopia, strabismus surgery should be delayed until maximal vision is obtained in the amblyopic eye.

For deprivation amblyopia induced by congenital cataract, the definitive treatment is surgery: removal of the cataract with or without intraocular lens (IOL) implantation. The age for IOL implantation in children is controversial. If the central cataract is less than 3 mm, surgery may not be necessary. However, these children must be examined and followed up frequently. If the cataract is dense and greater than 3 mm, prompt surgical removal is indicated during the first 6 weeks of life. If dense cataracts occur in both eyes, an interval of only several weeks between surgeries is indicated. If already started, patching therapy should be resumed after the cataract surgery until the visual acuity in both eyes becomes equal.

The first line of treatment for glaucoma-induced deprivation amblyopia is medical control (eye drops) of the IOP. If glaucoma medications fail to control the IOP and the progression of disease, surgical treatment (including goniotomy or filtering procedures) is warranted.

For deprivation amblyopia caused by corneal disorders, the primary treatment for corneal infection is medical (antibiotics). For severe scarring, corneal transplant surgery may be indicated.

In all forms of amblyopia, occlusion of the sound eye should be started before any other treatment—medical or surgical—and resumed after treatment.

References

1. Haider S, Qureshi W, Ali A. Leukocoria in children. *J Pediatr Strabismus*. 2008;45(3):179-180.
2. Shields CL, Gorry T, Shields JA. Outcome of eyes with unilateral sporadic retinoblastoma based on the initial external findings by the family and the pediatrician. *J Pediatr Strabismus*. 2004;41(3):143-149.

Suggested Readings

Amblyopia. In: *American Academy of Ophthalmology, Basic and Clinical Sciences Course.* Section 6: Pediatric Ophthalmology and Strabismus. San Francisco, CA: AAO; 2010-2011:61-67.

Drews-Botsch CD, Celano M, Kruger S, Hartman EE. Adherence to occlusion therapy in the first six months of follow-up and visual acuity among participants in the infant aphakia treatment study (IATS). *Invest Ophthalmol Vis Sci.* 2012;53(70):3368-3375.

Harley RD, Nelson, LB, Olitsky SE. *Harley's Pediatric Ophthalmology.* Philadelphia, PA: Lippincott Williams & Wilkins; 2005.

Plager DA, Lynn ML, Buckley EG, Wilson ME, Lambert SR. Complications, adverse events and additional intraocular surgery one year after cataract surgery in the infant aphakia treatment study. *Ophthalmology.* 2011;11(12):2330-2334.

WHAT SHOULD THE MEDICAL WORK-UP OF A BABY WITH CONGENITAL CATARACTS INCLUDE?

Dawn Duss, MD

The most critical point in evaluating a child with congenital cataracts is distinguishing between bilateral and unilateral involvement. Bilateral cataracts are often inherited or associated with systemic disease. Unilateral cataracts commonly arise from focal intraocular dysgenesis and are not associated with metabolic or syndromic abnormalities.

For bilateral cataracts, a hereditary or systemic association is generally identified in 60% to 70% of cases. Bilateral cataracts can be inherited in an autosomal-dominant (most common), autosomal-recessive, or X-linked manner, so a careful family history is critical and can avoid a costly work-up. Parents and siblings should be examined for clinically insignificant lens opacities because phenotypic variability is common, especially in autosomal-dominant cases. A history of febrile illness during pregnancy may suggest an infectious etiology such as Toxoplasmosis, Rubella, Cytomegalovirus, or Herpes simplex virus (TORCH) and prompt testing for antibody titers and subspecialty consultation.

Metabolic disorders, such as galactosemia, Fabry disease, and Wilson disease, are classically associated with morphologically distinct lens changes. Lens opacities in galactosemia occur in the posterior lens cortex and resemble an oil droplet on retroillumination. These opacities may regress with adequate dietary control. Wilson disease cataracts bear likeness to a sunflower, characterized by golden copper deposits on the anterior lens capsule. Renal disease, including Lowe and Alport's syndromes, may be associated with lens opacities that are discoid or located in the anterior subcapsular space, respectively. Christmas tree cataracts are seen in patients with myotonic dystrophy. Children with metabolic disorders may have characteristic physical features, such as frontal bossing and chubby cheeks (Lowe syndrome), tendon xanthomas (Wilson disease) or hepatomegaly (galactosemia). Careful physical examination by a pediatrician can help narrow the differential diagnosis.

Wagner RS. *Curbside Consultation in Pediatric*
Ophthalmology: 49 Clinical Questions (pp 47-50)
© 2014 SLACK Incorporated

Figure 9-1. (A) Persistent hyperplastic primary vitreous (PHPV) cataract presenting with a white pupil at birth. (B) Dense, vascular retrolental PHPV plaque with elongated ciliary processes.

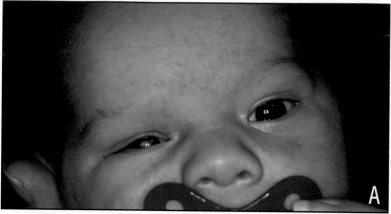

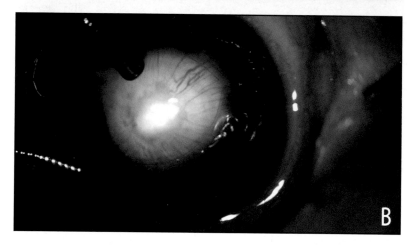

Bilateral congenital cataracts have been linked to a large number of chromosomal, craniofacial, and dermatological syndromes as well. Studies have shown a high incidence of cataracts in trisomy 21 patients, approaching 20%.[1] Onset may be delayed until late childhood, and many of these cataracts remain visually insignificant over time. Smith-Lemli-Opitz, Rubenstein-Taybi, Pierre Robin, and Crouzon syndromes also carry an increased risk of congenital cataracts.

Most unilateral pediatric cataracts are of unknown etiology, developing as a result of localized ocular dysgenesis. The most common types of unilateral cataract include persistent hyperplastic primary vitreous (PHPV), posterior lenticonus, and polar cataracts, both anterior and posterior. Other intraocular abnormalities may coexist, including microcornea, iris and angle anomalies, and posterior segment pathology. Stretched ciliary bodies and prominent iris blood vessels are commonly seen in cases of PHPV. Lens cortex may become spontaneously reabsorbed, leading to fusion of anterior and posterior capsule leaflets, in close union with a dense retrolental membrane (Figure 9-1). A complete dilated ophthalmic examination is recommended in all children with any type of congenital lens opacity. B-scan ultrasonography may be necessary in cases where view of the posterior pole is inadequate.

Visual prognosis varies with cataract morphology, and certain lens features may guide management protocols. Total, Morgagnian and membranous cataracts deprive a newborn of visual stimulus and can profoundly affect visual prognosis. Surgery must be completed before 6 to 8 weeks of age for best visual outcome (Figure 9-2). Other cataracts, such as lamellar, sutural, pulverulent (composed of tiny dots), and cerulean (blue or green in hue), rarely progress to become visually

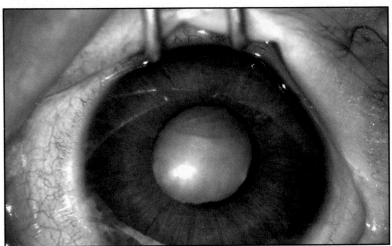

Figure 9-2. Total congenital cataract.

significant and can be monitored clinically in many cases. Anterior polar cataracts, likewise, may remain stable in appearance. Although they are generally small in size, they may induce significant refractive error, leading to anisometropia and subsequent amblyopia. Posterior lenticonus-type cataracts derive from focal thinning of the posterior lens capsule, with progressive bowing and distortion of lens fibers (Figure 9-3). Opacification of lens lamellae in this area can be rapidly progressive, necessitating surgical intervention. Even without opacification, posterior lenticonus may induce significant amounts of astigmatism. Close monitoring is recommended, especially in younger children who may not articulate changes in acuity. Monocular Teller acuity testing may be helpful in infants, and prophylactic amblyopia therapy can be considered.

For both bilateral and unilateral congenital cataracts, a detailed history including onset, family history, and developmental milestones is imperative. Exposure to radiation, chronic steroid use, or history of trauma should also be documented. For unilateral cataracts with morphology consistent with PHPV or posterior lenticonus, I do not generally perform an extensive work-up. Likewise, if a clear familial inheritance pattern is documented, comprehensive systemic evaluation may be deferred. For atypical unilateral or bilateral cataracts, I recommend a complete physical examination, genetics consultation, and laboratory studies. Laboratory studies include TORCH titers immunoglobulin m, rapid plasma regain, venereal disease research laboratory test, red cell galactokinase, galactose 1-phosphate uridyl transferase, serum calcium, serum phosphorus, and basic chemistry panel. I also obtain urine for amino acids and reducing substances after milk feeding. Obtaining urine studies in a neonate can be challenging and requires cooperation with the child's pediatrician. Spot urine testing may be adequate for amino acid evaluation; confirm with your local laboratory before pursuing 24-hour collection.

Figure 9-3. (A) Posterior lenticonus cataract. Bowing of posterior capsule with focal opacification. (B) Posterior lenticonus defect on retroillumination.

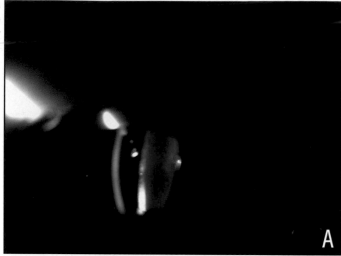

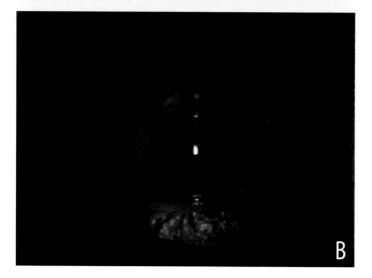

Reference

1. Wright KW. Lens abnormalities. In: Wright KW, Spiegel PH, eds. *Pediatric Ophthalmology and Strabismus.* 2nd ed. New York, NY: Springer-Verlag; 2003:450-480.

Suggested Readings

Amaya L, Taylor D, Russell-Eggit I, Nischal KK, Lengyel D. The morphology and natural history of childhood cataracts. *Surv Ophthalmol.* 2003;48(2):125-144.

Lambert SR. Cataract and persistent hyperplastic primary vitreous (PHPV). In: Taylor D, Hoyt CS, eds. *Pediatric Ophthalmology and Strabismus.* 3rd ed. Philadelphia, PA: Elsevier Saunders; 2005:441-457.

Lambert SR, Lynn MJ, Peeves R, Plager DA, Buckley EG, Wilson ME. Is there a latent period for the surgical treatment of children with dense bilateral cataracts? *J AAPOS.* 2006;10:30-36.

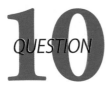

DO SYSTEMIC STEROIDS CAUSE OCULAR DISEASE? IF SO, UNDER WHAT CONDITIONS? HOW ABOUT INHALED STEROIDS?

Nina Ni, MD and Suqin Guo, MD

The ocular diseases most commonly manifested after use of topical, systemic, or inhaled corticosteroids (steroids) are cataract and glaucoma. Systemic steroids are commonly used for the treatment of airway diseases such as asthma, skin disorders, allergic reactions, and eczema in children.

Cataract is the leading cause of blindness worldwide, with surgery being the only effective treatment. Although the most common cause of cataract is aging, the use of systemic or ocular corticosteroids is a significant risk factor for the development of cataract. With steroid use, several factors come into play, including advanced age, patient's susceptibility to steroids, dosage, and duration of use.[1] The most common form of steroid-induced cataract is posterior subcapsular cataract. For both systemic and topically applied steroids, high dosages and prolonged periods of use are associated with a high incidence of posterior subcapsular cataract. Steroid-induced cataract is rare among children and is sometimes reversible after discontinuation of steroids.

A typical corticosteroid-induced cataract is characterized by subcapsular opacification located predominantly at the posterior cortical layers of the lens. This type of cataract is often axial and more visually disturbing than other types of cataract during the early course of the disease. Common complaints from the patient with posterior subcapsular cataract are glare and monocular double vision. These symptoms are worse under bright conditions, such as when reading or driving at night with oncoming headlights. This is primarily due to accommodation and light-induced miosis (ie, pupillary constriction under bright lighting), leading to more impaired visual acuity at near (reading) distances.

Glaucoma, a potentially blinding disease typified by high intraocular pressure (IOP), induces damage to the optic nerve head and causes loss of peripheral vision. Steroid-response glaucoma is known to be related to topical application of steroids (ie, drops and ocular injection). Glaucoma can also occur from systemic steroid use, although less frequently than from topical administration.

Wagner RS. *Curbside Consultation in Pediatric*
Ophthalmology: 49 Clinical Questions (pp 51-53)
© 2014 SLACK Incorporated

A patient may be predisposed to this condition if there is a positive family history of glaucoma, high myopia, or a previous diagnosis of glaucoma. Therefore, it is important to take a detailed medical history because family history of glaucoma and previous IOP problems provide invaluable diagnostic information.

In steroid-response glaucoma, you will typically see an early elevation of IOP within several days to several months after initiation of treatment. Dosage and duration of steroid use are also determining factors in steroid-response glaucoma. Thus, IOP measurement and complete eye examinations, including optic nerve and peripheral visual field testing, are critical for diagnosis. A study of 5 children with acute lymphoblastic leukemia, all of whom received oral or intravenous dexamethasone for 2.5 to 3 years, revealed that all 5 children developed ocular hypertension, which was well controlled with glaucoma medications.[2]

What Treatments Are Recommended?

Currently, there are no medical treatments for cataract. Surgery is the only effective treatment for steroid-induced and all other types of cataract. Cataract extraction with intraocular lens implantation has become a well-accepted standard of care procedure for children aged 2 years or older. The age for intraocular lens implantation in infants is still controversial due to higher surgical complication rates and the fast rate of growth of infants' eyes. Complications after cataract extraction surgery are different in children than in adults; for example, the risk of glaucoma is higher after cataract surgery in pediatric patients. It is therefore crucial to perform periodic eye examination and IOP measurement after surgery. Amblyopia treatment should be considered before and soon after cataract extraction surgery in young children.

For steroid-response glaucoma, discontinuation of use or reduction of dosage and frequency of steroid application are recommended as initial and most effective treatments. Changing to less potent steroids may also be helpful. In most cases, IOP returns to baseline levels after discontinuation of steroid use. Few patients will require surgical treatment when IOP is dangerously high and uncontrollable.

How About Inhaled Steroids?

For the past decade, inhaled corticosteroids (ICS) have been used to treat asthma, because they permit drug delivery to the lungs while minimizing systemic exposure.[3] Reports indicate that high doses of ICS not only increase the risk of cataract, glaucoma, and skin atrophy but also produce osteoporosis.

The association between cataract and ICS is related to higher inhaled doses. A study of more than 15,000 cataract patients revealed an increased risk for cataract with ICS use, compounded by high dosages, long duration of use, and older age.[1] With advancements in cataract surgical techniques and the resulting low associated morbidity, the potential benefits from control of pulmonary disease may outweigh the risk of cataract development. Nonetheless, given that high dosage and long duration of ICS use are associated with increased risk of cataract development, we recommend using the lowest dosage of ICS compatible with control of airway disease.

Fortunately for pediatricians, prolonged exposure to ICS increases the risk for subcapsular and nuclear cataracts more in older patients than in younger asthmatics.[2] A recent study of 266 asthmatic children (aged 7 to 11 years) treated with inhaled fluticacasone propionate spray for 3 to 6 years showed that no child developed any ocular adverse effects, including cataract, ocular hypertension, or glaucoma.[4] Generally speaking, long-term use and medium dosages of ICS do not increase the risk of cataracts in children and young adults.[4,5]

References

1. Smeeth L, Boulis M, Hubbard R, Fletcher AE. A population based case-control study of cataract and inhaled corticosteroids. *Br J Ophthalmol.* 2003;87:1247-1251.
2. Yamashita T, Kodama Y, Tanaka M, Yamakiri K, Kawano Y, Sakamoto T. Steroid-induced glaucoma in children with acute lymphoblastic leukemia: a possible complication. *J Glaucoma.* 2010;19(3):188-190.
3. Allen DB, Bielory L, Derendorf H, Dluhy R, Colice GL, Szefler SJ. Inhaled corticosteroids: past lessons and future issues. *J Allergy Clin Immunol.* 2003;112(3 suppl):S1-S40.
4. Emin O, Faith M, Mustafa O, Nedim S, Asman C. Evaluation impact of long-term usage of inhaled fluticasone propionate on ocular functions in children with asthma. *Steroids.* 2011;76(6):548-552.
5. Stoloff SW, Kelly HW. Updates on the use of inhaled corticosteroids in asthma. *Surr Opin Allergy Clin Immunol.* 2011;11(4):337-344.

SECTION III

TRAUMA

How Do I Diagnose and Treat Corneal Abrasions? Does Patching Remain an Important Component of Therapy?

Denise Hug, MD

Corneal abrasion is a common occurrence in children, and it is often initially diagnosed by the primary care provider.

As with almost everything in medicine, the diagnosis begins with history. Pertinent questions to be answered are mechanism of injury, offending material, and use of contact lenses. The mechanism of injury can be an important clue to the extent of injury. If the injury is a result of a high-velocity projectile, more severe injury such as a corneal laceration may be present. Corneal abrasions caused by paper, fingernails, and organic matter have been associated with recurrence.[1] Contact lens use, fingernail and organic matter injury are also more concerning for the development of infectious keratitis. Unfortunately, sometimes there is no history. This is particularly true for babies and toddlers, where an injury may not have been witnessed. Older children may be less than forthcoming when reporting the mechanism of injury because they are afraid to get in trouble. In verbal children, the most common complaint is that of pain followed by photophobia, eye redness, and tearing.[2] In preverbal children and infants, the patient may just present with crying, irritability, eye rubbing, and redness.[3]

Diagnosis

The physical examination to diagnose corneal abrasion is straightforward. Start with visual acuity in verbal children. The visual acuity may be significantly affected because of the disruption of the epithelial surface. Next, observe the anterior segment. The eyelid may be slightly red or puffy. The conjunctiva is usually injected. The epithelial defect can occasionally be seen with just the direct ophthalmoscope as an irregularity of the normally smooth surface. The key to

Wagner RS. *Curbside Consultation in Pediatric Ophthalmology: 49 Clinical Questions* (pp 57-60)
© 2014 SLACK Incorporated

Figure 11-1. Large central corneal abrasion staining with fluorescein. Notice the edge of the epithelium and how the dye has expanded into the adjacent cornea.

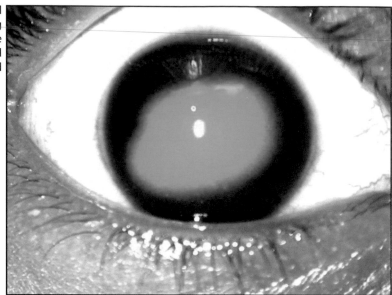

Figure 11-2. Linear corneal abrasion staining with fluorescein.

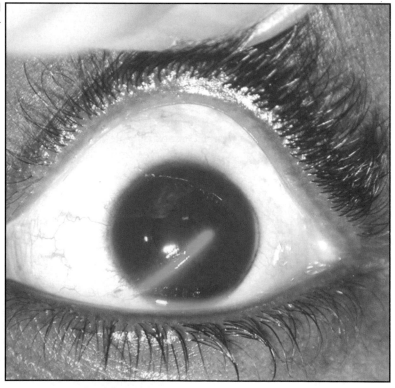

diagnosis is fluorescein staining of the cornea. Place a drop of fluorescein on the cornea and view the corneal surface with the direct ophthalmoscope that has a blue filter. If an abrasion is present, it will be bright green (Figures 11-1 and 11-2). A few caveats: use tetracaine early in the examination to facilitate getting a visual acuity and adequate examination. If the corneal abrasion is very large, involving almost the entire cornea, it is easy to miss because there is no normal cornea with which it can be compared. If the whole cornea is green, consider that the whole cornea is missing its epithelium. A Wood's lamp is a good way to look for corneal abrasions. It gives a large field of blue and highlights the epithelial defect well.

The diagnosis of corneal abrasion is made clinically and is usually straightforward. Occasionally, herpes virus keratitis may be confused as a corneal abrasion. The staining appearance of the cornea between them is different but in certain cases may be subtle. The classic appearance of herpes keratitis is that of a tree branch, which earned its name as a dendrite. As a corneal abrasion heals, it can take on a dendritic appearance. The important difference between the two is the history. Patients with herpes keratitis often present with a red, painful, photophobic eye that has been present for days with no history of known trauma. The other condition that should be considered is a corneal infiltrate or ulcer, especially if the patient is a contact lens wearer. These patients usually present with an acutely red, painful, photophobic eye. The infiltrate/ulcer may be located anywhere on the cornea but is often central or under the eyelid. A corneal ulcer will stain with fluorescein. The area of the infiltrate is white and fluffy. The area around the ulcer is also often white and elevated.

Treatment

Once the diagnosis of corneal abrasion is made, treatment is directed at keeping the child as comfortable as possible and healing the epithelial defect quickly and without infection. The cornea is well innervated and corneal abrasions are exquisitely painful, so it is difficult to control this particular pain. The best way to relieve the pain is to get the cornea re-epithelialized quickly. Acetaminophen and ibuprofen may be used to help with pain control. Narcotics may be used judiciously for pain control. Narcotics do not usually completely control the pain, but the biggest benefit of narcotics is sedation. Corneal abrasions tend to heal quickly, and if the child sleeps through most of the healing time, all the better. Cycloplegic agents such as cyclopentolate 1%, homatropine 2% or 5%, or atropine 1% should also be used for pain control. Photophobia is caused by the pupil constricting when exposed to light. By using dilating agents, the iris sphincter muscle is immobilized and the patient is more comfortable. The agent used depends on practitioner preference. Atropine has the advantage of having longer duration of action and does not sting quite as much. Parents should be warned, however, that there will be reduced near vision during therapy and for a few days following cessation of atropine drops. Topical antibiotic ointment should be used for infection prophylaxis and lubrication, which in turn improves comfort and promotes healing of the epithelium. There is no consensus on which antibiotic should be used. Available topical ophthalmic ointments include erythromycin, ciprofloxacin, tobramycin, and gentamicin.

The most controversial part of treating a corneal abrasion is whether to patch or not to patch. In the adult population, it has been shown that patching did not improve healing time, but there is still no consensus in the pediatric population. Michael et al[4] performed a study looking at healing rate, pain, and effect on activities of daily living comparing patching versus no patching in the treatment of corneal abrasion. The study showed no statistical difference in healing rate and pain. There was a difference in ambulation, which was more affected in the patching group. Because of these results, it is often recommended to use antibiotic ointment 4 to 6 times a day without patching. Patching may still be appropriate if the child is continuously rubbing the eye. If the patient is patched and removes the patch, initiate ophthalmic ointment 4 to 6 times daily.

Two final recommendations follow. First, do not use a topical steroid in the treatment of corneal abrasion. This includes the combination drugs such as Tobradex (tobramycin and dexamethasone) or Maxitrol (neomycin, polymyxin B sulfates, and dexamethasone). Second, never allow the patient to leave with tetracaine. Tetracaine is toxic to the epithelium and delays healing, which increases the duration of pain. This leads to increased use of the tetracaine, and a vicious cycle starts that can lead to corneal scar, permanent loss of vision, perforation of the cornea, and even loss of the eye.

Follow-up should occur 24 to 48 hours after initiation of treatment. The follow-up may be performed by the primary caregiver if he or she is comfortable managing the corneal abrasion. If not, the patient should be directed to an ophthalmologist for ongoing treatment. Once the patient is comfortable, the cycloplegic agent may be discontinued. Once the epithelial defect is resolved, the ointment may be discontinued.

My personal recommendation includes atropine 1% 1 drop 2 times daily, erythromycin ophthalmic ointment 6 times daily, and nonnarcotic analgesics. If the patient is a contact lens wearer or the injury was from organic material or fingernail, use ciprofloxacin ointment instead of the erythromycin. My preference is not to patch unless the child continues to rub the eye. Even very large abrasions heal well without patching, and patching has not been shown to improve healing rates even in these large abrasions. Once the epithelial defect is resolved, I usually continue the ointment for an additional 3 to 7 days in hopes of decreasing the possibility of recurrence. When we sleep, the cornea swells slightly, and if the epithelium is not well-adhered to the underlying layer of cornea, the epithelium may be sloughed off when the child opens his or her eyelid in the morning. By lubricating the cornea at bedtime for an extra few days, it allows time for the adherence of the epithelium to improve. If the abrasion is large, it takes a bit more time to adhere, so continue the ointment for the full 7 days.

References

1. Weene LE. Recurrent corneal erosion after trauma: a statistical study. *Ann Ophthalmol.* 1985;17:521-524.
2. Butler HB, Reisdorff EJ. The red eye: a systematic approach to differential diagnosis and therapy. *Emerg Med Rep.* 1994;15:43-52.
3. Harkness MJ. Corneal abrasion in infancy as a cause of inconsolable crying. *Pediatr Emerg Care.* 1989;5:242-244.
4. Michael JG, Hug D, Dowd MD. Management of corneal abrasion in children: a randomized clinical trial. *Ann Emerg Med.* 2002;40:67-72.

HOW DO I MANAGE CORNEAL AND CONJUNCTIVAL FOREIGN BODIES?

William Constad, MD

Conjunctival and corneal foreign bodies are fairly common causes of ocular complaints. Most of the time they are easily treated by the primary care physician, but care must be taken not to miss a more serious injury that could lead to serious complications and even loss of sight. Diagnosing either of these conditions is more difficult in children because you may have a nonverbal or unco-operative historian. Often you will be faced with a child who won't voluntarily open the eye and has tearing and light sensitivity. The application of a topical anesthetic drop as described next will go a long way in allowing you to perform an examination because, as pain relief may be instanta-neous. Always be suspicious of a foreign body or corneal abrasion when faced with a patient with one eye that is painful and inflamed while the other eye is without symptoms.

What you may need:

- Bottle of topical anesthetic, such as tetracaine or proparacaine. In a pinch, a drop or 2 of inject-able lidocaine 1% or 2% can be used. The injectable form is not buffered for topical use and may sting for a short time until the anesthetic takes effect.

- A few sterile applicator sticks

- Fluorescein strips

- Some sterile balanced salt solution, or eye wash solution

- Cobalt blue light, or at least a good penlight

Wagner RS. *Curbside Consultation in Pediatric Ophthalmology: 49 Clinical Questions* (pp 61-64)
© 2014 SLACK Incorporated

Figure 12-1. Note that the applicator tip is placed above the lashes in the fold of the lid. Grasp the eyelashes, lift them, and fold the lid over the tip of the applicator.

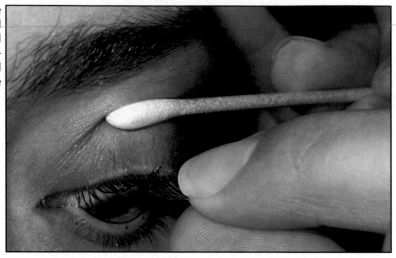

Conjunctival Foreign Bodies

A foreign body on the conjunctiva can either be insidious or symptomatic. The degree of symptoms and clinical signs will depend on the size, location, and material of the foreign body.

The conjunctiva can be separated anatomically into 2 general regions, referred to as the bulbar conjunctiva and the palpebral conjunctiva. The bulbar conjunctiva covers the anterior surface of the eyeball, beginning at the edge of the cornea and extending to the superior and inferior fornices, where the conjunctiva then reflects over itself and onto the inner surface of the eyelid, where it is referred to as the palpebral conjunctiva.

A foreign body on the bulbar conjunctiva can sometimes be seen easily, but it may be necessary to gently pull down the lower eyelid. The conjunctiva surrounding the foreign body will likely be injected. Surface foreign bodies can often be easily removed by first using a drop of topical anesthetic, then gently irrigating with balanced salt solution or a stream from an eye wash bottle. If the foreign body is more adherent, you can gently wipe it with an applicator stick. Do not press hard or wipe firmly; if the foreign body has penetrated the conjunctiva, it may get pushed through and more injury can be inflicted with pressure. If the patient complains of a foreign body sensation and no foreign body is visible, you can often evert the upper eyelid by placing an applicator stick horizontally across the fold of the upper lid (Figure 12-1), lifting the lashes, and folding the upper lid over the applicator stick (Figure 12-2). You may see a foreign body stuck to the underside of the lid (called the tarsal surface). This can usually be removed by gently wiping with another applicator stick. Sometimes the foreign body can be extremely small, although quite symptomatic (Figure 12-3).

A clue to the presence of a foreign body on the undersurface of the upper lid is vertical corneal abrasions (see Figure 11-2). If you cannot remove the foreign body, instill an ophthalmic antibiotic ointment and refer to an ophthalmologist. As well, if there is evidence of a conjunctival laceration, which might be suggested by the presence of a subconjunctival hemorrhage, refer to an ophthalmologist.

Some of the complications associated with conjunctival foreign bodies are related, not only to the physical size and shape but to material as well. For instance, it is not uncommon to have particles of gypsum (from sheet rock) get into the inferior cul-de-sac. One of the major ingredients of sheet rock is lime. This can cause a chemical burn, which can cause permanent damage if not

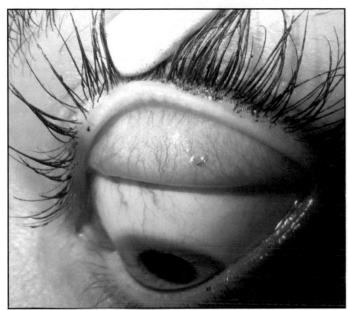

Figure 12-2. With the lid folded back, you should be able to slide the applicator stick out of the fold and place on top of the eyelashes to hold the lid in position. In this case, you can see the foreign body on the upper tarsus. The foreign body can be gently wiped off the upper tarsus with a sterile applicator.

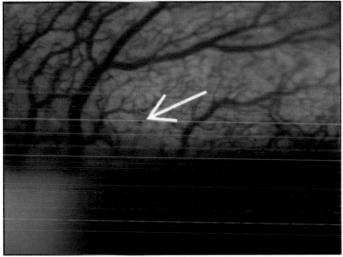

Figure 12-3. If you look carefully, you can see a small foreign body. Even a foreign body this small can cause symptoms.

removed and irrigated quickly. Organic matter can cause a lot of inflammation and can also be a vector for fungal infections.

Corneal Foreign Bodies

Corneal foreign bodies tend to be symptomatic, with the patient reporting tearing, burning, photophobia, blurry vision, foreign body sensation, and pain. Sometimes children present with an unrecognized foreign body after having a "red eye" for a few days that is not resolving. Careful inspection of the cornea with a penlight may reveal a small foreign body imbedded in the cornea (Figure 12-4).

Figure 12-4. Small, metallic foreign body embedded in the cornea with a small rust ring surrounding. While you may attempt to irrigate this, it may be necessary to refer the patient to an ophthalmologist.

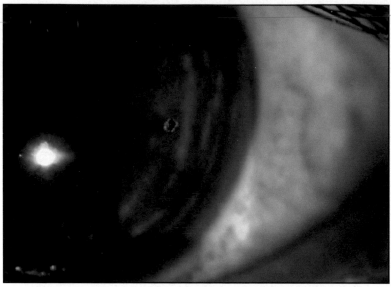

The cornea is the clear layer of tissue that functions as the first lens of the eye. Sixty percent of the focusing power of the eye comes from the cornea. If the corneal surface is irregular, dry, or scarred; if there is swelling in the cornea or if there is any haze in the cornea, the vision can be dramatically affected. The cornea is made up of layers of collagen lamellae that are organized in parallel layers, much like an onion skin. Any disturbance of this parallel arrangement of cells causes decreased vision.

If a foreign body has been present in the cornea for a while and is small enough to lie flat on the surface, some of the patient's initial symptoms may lessen as mucus adheres to the surface of the foreign body, masking some of the more annoying symptoms. The major concerns with foreign bodies on the cornea are infection and penetration. Normal corneal thickness is in the range of 500 to 550 microns, so if a foreign body is sharp or pointy and strikes the cornea with sufficient velocity, it can penetrate the cornea or embed itself deeply. Corneal foreign bodies should be removed after instillation of topical anesthetic and only by irrigation. If it cannot be removed with irrigation, refer to an ophthalmologist.

Foreign bodies such as glass and plastic can sometimes be difficult to see. These materials will often have sharp edges that can penetrate the conjunctiva, cornea, and wall of the eye. If there is any question of penetration through the conjunctiva or deeper, immediate referral to an ophthalmologist is required.

Following the removal of a corneal foreign body, there may be a residual corneal abrasion. These are usually managed with topical ophthalmic antibiotic ointments or drops. Large abrasions may require a pressure patch.

Suggested Readings

American Academy of Ophthalmology Web site. http://www.aao.org/theeyeshaveit/trauma/foreignbody-corneal. cfm. Accessed February 2, 2014.

Feied C, Smith M, Handler J, Gillam M. NCEMI Web site. http://www.ncemi.org/cse/cse0204.htm. Accessed February 2, 2014.

Klyce SD, Beuerman RW. Structure and function of the cornea. In: Kaufman HE, Barron BA, McDonald MB, et al. *The Cornea*. New York, NY: Churchill Livingstone; 1988:3-54.

HOW CAN I RECOGNIZE A PERFORATING OCULAR INJURY?

Ronald Rescigno, MD

Initially, it is important to ascertain a complete account of the accident. This is not accomplished easily in a young preverbal child following an accidental or other type of ocular trauma. You may be faced initially with a crying child forcefully closing the injured eye. You should attempt to get the eyelids open to at least inspect the integrity of the globe. A drop of a topical anesthetic into the eye may prove useful. It is important to understand that there are 2 types of injuries that may cause a ruptured eye.

The first type of injury is a perforation of the cornea and/or anterior sclera. This type of injury in the pediatric population usually occurs by pencils, scissors, darts, or other sharp objects.

The second type of injury is caused by blunt trauma to the eye. The anterior-posterior dimensions of the eye get compressed, and the weakest part of the sclera gets ruptured. This type of injury occurs behind the extraocular muscles, which are 5 to 6 mm behind the corneal-scleral limbus. This happens because the sclera is thinnest behind the eye muscles. Injuries like this can occur when a hockey puck or a paintball hits the eye without proper eye protection.

The perforation type of injury is the easiest to evaluate on clinical examination. If a sharp object perforates the cornea, there are several findings that you may see on your examination. The visual acuity in these patients can range from normal to poor. Start with the easiest and move to the more difficult. If you see a corneal injury, with iris to the corneal wound (Figure 13-1), a flat anterior chamber (from leakage of aqueous humor), and a white lens (traumatic cataract happens rapidly when the anterior capsule of the lens is penetrated), the eye is ruptured. The other extreme is the full-thickness corneal laceration, where there is no iris to the wound or cataract and a formed or shallow anterior chamber. The patient usually has good visual acuity. For this type of injury, you need a slit lamp and fluorescein strips. Wipe the area of the corneal injury with a fluorescein strip and look at the same time with the cobalt blue light on a slit lamp (Seidel test). You will initially see

Wagner RS. *Curbside Consultation in Pediatric Ophthalmology: 49 Clinical Questions* (pp 65-67)
© 2014 SLACK Incorporated

Figure 13-1. Iris incarcerated in the cornea with peaked pupil toward the laceration.

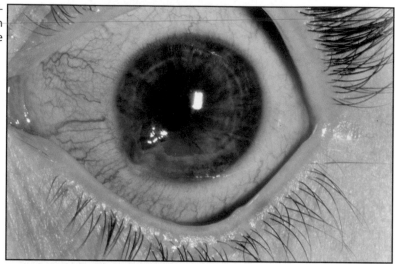

Figure 13-2. Scleral laceration with uveal prolapse, peaked pupil, and hyphema. The area of the rupture is clear because there is no hemorrhagic chemosis.

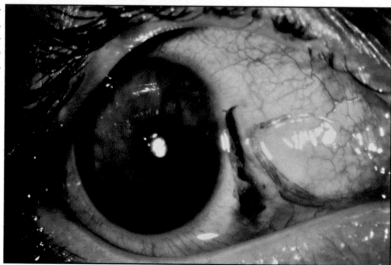

a dark orange color, and if the cornea is leaking, you will see a stream of light green flowing down the cornea. This phenomenon occurs because as the fluorescein gets diluted from aqueous humor, it lightens to a green color. Place a shield on the eye and refer immediately to an ophthalmologist. If you don't have an eye shield, you can cut a small paper cup in half and tape it over the eye.

The other type of anterior segment perforating injury to the eye involves the anterior sclera (Figure 13-2). Let's say a child is hit with a sharp object in the sclera not involving the cornea, the cornea does not stain with fluorescein, and there is an area of hemorrhagic chemosis where the object hit (looking like a swollen subconjunctival hemorrhage with swelling of the conjunctiva). Is this a conjunctival hemorrhage or a perforating ocular injury? What you want to look for here is the pupil. If the pupil is irregular and peaked toward the area of hemorrhage, I would suspect a scleral laceration, and refer as described previously.

The blunt ocular injury is more difficult to evaluate. These types of injuries uniformly have poor visual acuity. Many of these injuries have diffuse hemorrhagic chemosis. In these types of injuries, hyphema (blood in the anterior chamber) and vitreous hemorrhage are commonly seen. The anterior chamber may appear to be deeper in posterior injuries, not shallow as in anterior injuries. If the patient has good vision, a posterior ruptured globe is unlikely. The best way to evaluate this type of injury is a computed tomography (CT) scan. On CT scan, the globe contour may look irregular or the globe may look disorganized. All types of perforating globe injuries usually have low intraocular pressure.

Although a pediatrician can initially manage certain types of ocular injuries such as corneal abrasions, other injuries should be immediately referred to an ophthalmologist. Hyphemas (especially in children with sickle-trait or sickle cell disease) can develop extremely high intraocular pressures. Also, potentially perforating ocular injuries as described above may require immediate surgery to repair the ocular laceration.

Suggested Readings

Pieramici DJ. Open globe injuries are rarely hopeless. *Review of Ophthalmology*. June 2005. Available at: http://www.revophth.com. Accessed April 27, 2012.

Pugh SM, Pasternak JF, Liszewski PA. Index of suspicion case 1. *Pediatr Rev.* 2010;31(7):303-307.

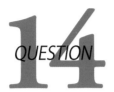

WHAT ARE THE SIGNS AND SYMPTOMS OF AN ORBITAL FRACTURE?

Roger E. Turbin, MD, FACS

Children with orbital fractures may present with signs and symptoms similar to those in adults. However, compared with their adult counterparts, children more commonly have clinically significant motility problems, despite more limited signs of bruising (white-eyed blowout[1]), and typically require earlier intervention to avoid permanent ocular misalignment. This discussion will be limited to the orbital floor fracture in the setting of limited facial trauma, rather than to more extensive closed head trauma or penetrating orbitocranial injury. More severe injuries predispose to complex fractures, including nasoethmoidal complex fractures, zygomatico-maxillary tripod fractures, skull base fractures involving the orbital canal, and Le Forte midfacial fractures. Penetrating injury also represents a topic with which clinicians ought to be familiar, given the difficulty and occasionally failure of computed tomography (CT) imaging to recognize orbitocranial penetration as well as occult foreign bodies composed of dry and hydrated wood. The latter two may have CT signal indistinguishable from air or surrounding tissue, respectively.

Orbital fractures in general occur due to direct disruption of the superior or inferior orbital rims, transmission of buckling forces to the orbital roof, floor or medial wall by blunt trauma, or indirect "globe to bone transmission of force" through hydraulic mechanisms, as well as any combination of these factors. Mechanical factors (thicker sinus walls, greater bone elasticity, more cheek fat pad, and a proportionately smaller and flatter midface) in children under the age of 7 years contribute to a relatively lower incidence of isolated orbital floor factures compared with older children and adults.[2] In this younger group, orbital roof fractures are more common.[3] In older children, orbital floor fractures become increasingly common and clinically important. In this entity, high relative tissue elasticity contributes to linear, hinged fractures that spring back into place and entrap peri orbital tissue or the inferior rectus muscle. The latter may rapidly cause extraocular muscle tissue ischemia, which may contribute to the inadequate postsurgical return of motility despite adequate bone and tissue reduction. However, in children, approximately 70% of orbital fractures are orbital floor fractures despite these trends.[4] With increasing age into adulthood, the less elastic orbital

Wagner R. *Curbside Consultation in Pediatric*
Ophthalmology: 49 Clinical Questions (pp 69-72)
© 2014 SLACK Incorporated

floor fractures result in more "open door" displacements of larger fracture fragments, which lead to less frequent ischemic muscle entrapment.

Symptoms of orbital fractures, the description of which may obviously be more difficult to elicit in the younger child, may include infraorbital or intraoral numbness or tingling, double or blurry vision, and gaze-induced pain or nausea. Children frequently experience pain, nausea, or vomiting with eye movement out of proportion to the degree of bruising. These findings are also highly suggestive of a clinically significant entrapped eye muscle or surrounding tissue. In the extreme case, the child may experience gaze-evoked vasovagal syncope due to bradycardia induced by the trigeminal–vagal—induced oculocardiac reflex.[5]

A complete examination of the eye and adnexa should include determination of best visual acuity (refraction or pinhole); assessment of the integrity of globe and anterior segment, presence of hyphema, and integrity of angle structures in cases of suspected anterior segment trauma; and dilated ophthalmoscopic examination. In the upset or anxious child, examination under anesthesia may be necessary. Clinical signs nearly conclusive for fracture include an area of hypoesthesia below the eye or superior intraoral gingival surface, subcutaneous orbital emphysema, enophthalmos, and characteristic patterns of ocular motility limitation. Careful attention to supraduction, infraduction, abduction, and adduction is paramount to recognition of entrapped orbital tissue. The presence of limited elevation in upgaze (supraduction) and restricted depression in downgaze (infraduction) is nearly pathognomic for a clinically significant orbital fracture with entrapment that likely demands rapid surgical attention.

Although CT remains the imaging procedure of choice in most situations, it frequently underestimates the extent of fracture and degree of tissue entrapment.[6] Radiographically, "trapdoor" blowout fractures may appear small but often severely limit ocular motility with entrapment of extraocular muscle, orbital connective tissue, or fat. In older patients and especially adults, decreasing bone and soft tissue elasticity contributes to larger fracture fragments, and often "open door" fractures with lower risk of entrapment. Orbital magnetic resonance imaging (MRI) imaging, which may require sedation in younger children, may have a selected role in special situations that require high-resolution soft tissue imaging or the elimination of radiographic exposure.

Ideally, surgery should not be performed on the basis of imaging alone but weigh both radiographic and clinical considerations that provide evidence of clinically significant fractures. Restrictive entrapment is a strong indicator for the need for timely surgical management. Suspicion of ocular muscle ischemia or bradycardic syncope signal a need for urgent intervention.

Case Presentation

A 4-year-old boy, elbowed by his brother, suffered a "white-eyed blowout" of the orbital floor with little sign of direct periocular bruising or facial trauma. The boy described position-dependant double vision and said his face felt funny. In primary gaze (Figure 14-1A), subtle enophthalmos is detectable, demonstrated by a deeper position of the affected right globe. Photographically less obvious than at clinical examination, the interpalpebral distance on the right was approximately 1.5 mm more narrow than the left, which also supports enophthalmos. In upgaze (Figure 14-1B), the elevation of the right eye is limited, and the eye is therefore hypotropic (Figure 14-1C). There is correspondingly less inferior scleral show between the lower eyelid and the limbus on the right. In downgaze, the depression of the right eye is limited, and the eye is hypertropic. There is correspondingly less superior scleral show on the right. A coronal CT scan of the orbit (Figure 14-2) shows a small fracture line adjacent to the infraorbital nerve, a common area of bone disruption. An intraoperative photograph (Figure 14-3) represents the fracture line after reduction of the entrapped tissue from his "trapdoor" prior to placement of a porous polyethylene orbital implant.

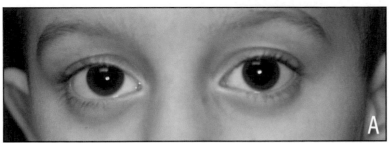

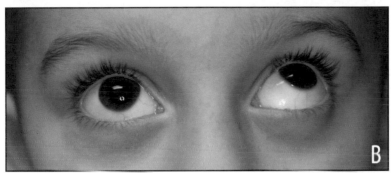

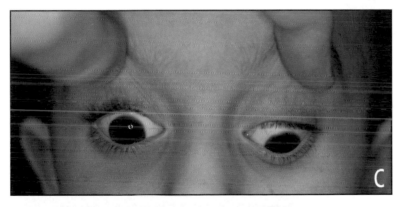

Figure 14-1. (A) Facial photograph of the child in primary gaze showing mild right enophthalmos with straight ocular alignment (orthotropia). (B) In upgaze, elevation is limited and the eye is hypotropic. (C) In downgaze, the eye depression is limited and the eye is hypertropic.

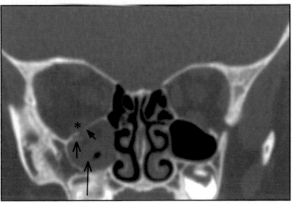

Figure 14-2. Coronal CT reconstruction of the orbits. In this image, a small fracture is imaged as a discontinuous segment of the right orbital floor (arrowhead) and a small fragment is present (short arrow), which probably represents a segment of the infraorbital canal. The inferior rectus is incarcerated in the hole (asterisk). The right maxillary sinus is full of blood and mucous (long arrow).

Figure 14-3. Intraoperative endoscopic photograph of the left orbital floor, viewed from the orbital side looking inferiorly at the bone defect of the orbital floor along the projection of the infraorbital nerve into the maxillary sinus below.

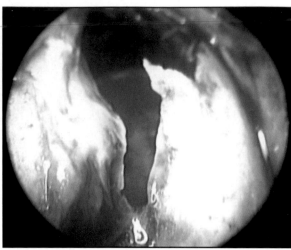

References

1. Jordan DR, Allen LH, White J, et al. Intervention within days for some orbital floor fractures: the white-eyed blowout. *Ophthal Plast Reconstr Surg.* 1998;14:379-390.
2. Koltai PJ, Amjad I, Meyer D, et al. Orbital fractures in children. *Arch Otolaryngol Head Neck Surg.* 1995;121:1375-1379.
3. Chapman VM, Fenton LZ, Gao D, et al. Facial fractures in children: unique patterns of injury observed by computed tomography. *J Comput Assist Tomogr.* 2009;33:70-72.
4. Wei LA, Durairaj VD. Pediatric orbital floor fractures. *J AAPOS.* 2011;15(2):173-180.
5. Sires BS, Stanley RB, Levine LM. Oculocardiac reflex caused by orbital floor trapdoor fracture: an indication for urgent repair. *Arch Ophthalmol.* 1998;116:955-956.
6. Parbhu KC, Galler KE, Li C, et al. Underestimation of soft tissue entrapment by computed tomography in orbital floor fractures in the pediatric population. *Ophthalmology.* 2008;115:1620-1625.

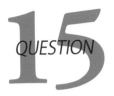
HOW DO I MANAGE A TRAUMATIC IRITIS?

Nina Ni, MD and Suqin Guo, MD

Traumatic iritis is inflammation of the iris—the anterior portion of the uvea that forms the pupil—caused by eye injury. Typically, patients with this entity present with a history of recent eye trauma (within a few days) and have eye pain, light sensitivity (photophobia), reduced visual acuity, and red eye. In many cases, the deep conjunctival and episcleral vascular injection causing the red eye will be localized primarily at the limbus. This "ciliary flush" is typical of intraocular inflammation in contrast to the diffuse vascular injection seen in cases of conjunctivitis. Concurrent subconjunctival hemorrhages can make this differentiation difficult. Symptoms worsen if light is shined into the traumatized eye or even into the other normal eye. The pressure inside the eye (the intraocular pressure) is either very high or very low.

Patients in whom traumatic iritis is suspected should be referred to an ophthalmologist, who will perform detailed eye examinations. Slit-lamp examination with a bright light beam will reveal white cells and glare in the anterior chamber. The pupil of the traumatized eye is usually small with irregular boundaries caused by traumatic tears in the iris sphincter muscles. There may also be scar formation (posterior synechiae) between the iris and lens capsule. Floating (microhyphema) or layered (hyphema) red blood cells may be present in the anterior chamber.

A number of complications are associated with traumatic iritis, including bleeding in the anterior chamber (traumatic hyphema), cataract, vitreous hemorrhage, retinal tears, or retinal detachment. It is vital to carefully examine both the anterior and posterior segments of the eye. Thus, a complete and thorough eye examination should be performed, including slit-lamp biomicroscopy for examination of the anterior segment of the eye and dilated ophthalmoscopy for examination of the optic nerve and retina. Special examination of the anterior chamber angle is important to detect any angle damage, which could predispose the eye to glaucoma. For the posterior segment,

Wagner R. *Curbside Consultation in Pediatric*
Ophthalmology: 49 Clinical Questions (pp 73-75)
© 2014 SLACK Incorporated

it is critical to check the retina to ensure that you are not missing a retinal detachment or an occult ruptured globe (which can be associated with any severe eye trauma) because these conditions require immediate surgical intervention.

Management of Traumatic Iritis and Associated Conditions

Management is similar to that of nontraumatic iritis (ie, iritis that is not caused by trauma, as may occur in cases of juvenile idiopathic arthritis). In both cases, most ophthalmologists treat with topical corticosteroids administered 3 to 4 times daily. Because the inflammation in this condition is often mild and self-limited, topical steroids with low potency and minimal effects on the intraocular pressure are recommended. For severe traumatic iritis, cycloplegic agents are often recommended because these will act to dilate the pupil, prevent scar formation, relax ciliary spasms, reduce photophobia, and lessen the eye pain resulting from inflammation. Miotic agents, which constrict the pupil, are contraindicated in patients with traumatic iritis because miotics can worsen inflammation and increase the risk of posterior synechiae formation. Elevated intraocular pressure (secondary glaucoma) can be associated with traumatic iritis due to direct injury to the chamber angle, inflammatory cells and debris clogging the chamber angle, or traumatic hyphema. Antiglaucoma medications should be administered if eye pressure is elevated.

Without proper treatment, traumatic iritis can lead to posterior synechiae, narrow-angle glaucoma, cataract, retinal/macular edema (which can cause severe loss of vision), or sympathetic ophthalmia.

Traumatic hyphema is often associated with traumatic iritis and deserves special consideration in children. Hyphema is characterized by intraocular bleeding with resulting accumulation of blood and clots in the anterior chamber. The most common cause of hyphema is eye trauma. A complete eye examination is mandated. If the blood in the anterior chamber obscures the view of the intraocular structures, B-scan ultrasound is necessary to rule out traumatic vitreous hemorrhage, retinal tear, retinal detachment, or occult open globe injury. Computed tomography (CT) scan of the orbit is required if an intraocular foreign body or a ruptured globe is suspected. Secondary glaucoma may result from both traumatic iritis and hyphema. Intraocular pressure should be measured and monitored regularly in patients with traumatic iritis and hyphema. Elevated eye pressure may be an indication for glaucoma therapy or a sign of recurrent hemorrhage during follow-up. Rebleeding of hyphema usually occurs within 1 week of the initial bleeding and increases the risk of secondary glaucoma. We also suggest that all children with traumatic hyphema be screened for sickle cell hemoglobinopathies, because these conditions are associated with higher incidence of rebleeding and secondary glaucoma. The principles of treatment for traumatic hyphema are similar to that of iritis, including topical corticosteroids to reduce inflammation and cycloplegic/mydriatic agents to decease ciliary spasm, photophobia, and the risk of posterior synechia formation. If eye pressure is high, aqueous suppressants, hyperosmotics, and carbonic anhydrase inhibitors are often administered. Carbonic anhydrase inhibitors should be avoided in children with sickle cell hemoglobinopathies due to the risk of metabolic acidosis. Prostaglandin agents should also be used with caution in all patients with iritis because these agents can aggravate inflammation.

Sympathetic ophthalmia is a rare, bilateral eye condition associated with a severe penetrating eye trauma to one eye. Because eye trauma may cause an autoimmune reaction to normally occult ocular tissue antigens, this response to itself can cause a panuveitis of the nontraumatized (normal) eye. In other words, bilateral inflammation of the iris and ciliary body (iridocyclitis) or choroid (choroiditis) may result from unilateral injury. You should always be highly suspicious of sympathetic ophthalmia in patients with a previous history of a penetrating injury to one eye and panuveitis of both eyes. These patients should be referred to an ophthalmologist immediately for treatment.

Conclusion

You should especially consider referring children with eye trauma to an ophthalmologist when they present with the following:

- Severe eye pain
- Photophobia
- Red eye
- Blood in the anterior chamber (hyphema)
- Reduced visual acuity
- Poor or asymmetrical red reflex in the pupils as seen by looking into both pupils using a direct ophthalmoscope (normal pupillary reflex should be bright and symmetrical in both eyes)

Suggested Readings

Acuna OM, Yen KG. Outcome and prognosis of pediatric patients with delayed diagnosis of open-globe injuries. *J Pediatr Ophthalmol Strabismus.* 2009;46(4):202-207.

Galea M, Falzon K, Chadha V, Williams G. Presumed occult globe rupture resulting in sympathetic ophthalmia. *J Ophthalmic Inflamm Infect.* 2012;2(3):137-140.

Meier P. Combined anterior and posterior segment injuries in children: a review. *Graefes Arch Clin Exp Ophthalmol.* 2010;248(9):1207 1219.

Podhielski DW, Surkont M, Tehrani NN, Ratnapalan S. Pediatric eye injuries in a Canadian emergency department. *Can J Ophthalmol.* 2009;44(5):519-522.

Walton W, Von Hagen S, Grigorian R, Zarbin M. Managements of traumatic hyphema. *Surv Ophthalmol.* 2002;47(4):297-334.

SHOULD I SUTURE EYELID LACERATIONS, OR CAN I USE GLUE?

Paul D. Langer, MD, FACS

Topical skin adhesives, or glues, are liquid cyanoacrylate derivatives that rapidly polymerize from monomers into long, solid chains upon contact with water. When these liquid monomers are placed on an open wound and react with the moisture in the skin, the resulting solid polymer strongly binds the skin edges together until healing occurs, thus replacing the function of sutures. The use of these adhesives to close superficial lacerations (or to close the skin portion of a deep wound in which the subdermal tissues have already been approximated with sutures) has become widespread since the US Food and Drug Administration approved the first such glue, Dermabond (Johnson & Johnson), in 1998.

Advantages

Skin adhesives possess several advantages over sutures in the closure of superficial lacerations, especially in the pediatric population. Placing the liquid over a laceration is quick, and the technique is comparatively easy and requires minimal training. The glue polymer itself forms a tight barrier over the wound that preserves the moist environment necessary for proper healing, and at the same time, prevents microbial penetration into the underlying tissue. Indeed, topical skin adhesives have been shown to possess antimicrobial activity in vitro, whereas sutures can actually serve as a nidus for infection.[1] Additionally, as natural wound healing occurs, the solid polymer sloughs, usually in 7 to 10 days, eliminating the additional psychological trauma and the difficulty of suture removal in a child. Finally, the cosmetic result of a wound closed with adhesives is the same as, or superior to, the cosmetic result of a wound closed with sutures, without an increase in the rate of wound dehiscence.[2,3]

Wagner R. *Curbside Consultation in Pediatric Ophthalmology: 49 Clinical Questions* (pp 77-80)
© 2014 SLACK Incorporated

Skin adhesives can be used to approximate many, but not all, eyelid lacerations. A basic familiarity with the properties of these adhesives, knowledge of the proper technique for their application, and an understanding of the appropriate lacerations for which they are indicated are all required prior to their use in the periocular area.

Two types of medical cyanoacrylates are currently in use: octyl cyanoacrylates (eg, Dermabond) and butyl cyanoacrylates (eg, Histoacryl; B. Braun Co). The difference in their chemical structures results in important physical properties that impact clinical use. Butyl cyanoacrylates, with a shorter side chain, polymerize more rapidly (within 30 seconds), but the resulting bonds are more brittle than with the octyl cyanoacrylates. Octyl cyanoacrylates, with a longer side chain, polymerize more slowly (over 2 to 3 minutes) but form bonds that are generally stronger and more flexible. For shorter wounds under low tension, clinical outcomes are generally similar when comparing the 2 types of adhesives, although there is some evidence that wounds under higher tension are less likely to dehisce following repair with octyl cyanoacrylates.[4]

Topical skin adhesives are ideally suited to close lacerations whose edges are easily approximated with minimal tension. Most authors recommend their use only in place of sutures that are size 5-0 or smaller. These adhesives work exceptionally well to close stellate or jagged lacerations as well as skin flaps because meticulous suturing of small and irregular borders is obviated once the lacerated skin edges are properly aligned.

How to Use Skin Adhesives

The technique for closing wounds with topical adhesives is straightforward. The wound should be copiously irrigated and cleaned, with povidone-iodine if necessary, and debridement performed if clinically indicated. Deeper wounds should have subcutaneous sutures placed so that the subsequent application of adhesive closes only the skin. The skin should then be dried, and the edges of the laceration temporarily held in apposition with forceps, surgical tape, finger pressure, or in some cases an assistant, while the adhesive is applied.

Octyl cyanoacrylates are applied across the wound in a linear fashion in 2 to 3 layers, waiting 30 seconds between each layer. The longer time for the octyl cyanoacrylates to polymerize allows the polymer to adhere in a multilayered matrix. Conversely, the butyl cyanoacrylates, which polymerize more quickly, are applied in a single layer because vertical bonding to a second layer cannot occur. Butyl cyanoacrylates, unlike their octyl counterparts, are applied in discrete drops across the length of the wound, like spot-welding.[5] Regardless of the type of glue used, adhesive should not be introduced into the wound because the presence of glue below the skin can delay healing and also cause discoloration (staining). Adhesive should therefore be applied gently over the wound without excess pressure. Should adhesive inadvertently be introduced into the wound, application of a topical antibiotic ointment will facilitate its removal.[5]

Following wound closure, no dressing or antibiotic ointment is necessary because the adhesive creates its own watertight, bacteriostatic cover. In fact, the use of antibiotic ointment should be discouraged because it may result in the adhesive becoming dislodged. Butyl cyanoacrylates should be kept dry for the first 48 hours after application, while octyl cyanoacrylates can be exposed to light moisture, such as showering. Neither type should be exposed to excessive water, such as in prolonged bathing or swimming, or premature sloughing of the polymer may occur.

If the above instructions are followed, topical skin adhesives can be an excellent alternative to sutures in the closure of pediatric eyelid lacerations. However, specific precautions in the use of topical adhesives around the eye should be noted. Although topical adhesives are not toxic to the surface of the eye (they have been used for years to close corneal perforations), it is still advisable to prevent adhesive from entering the palpebral aperture to avoid the eyelids and/or lashes from

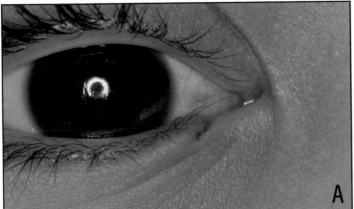

Figure 16-1. Repairing marginal eyelid lacerations with adhesives is not recommended. (A) Small eyelid laceration in a child involving the medial aspect of the right lower eyelid. (B) Everting the eyelid reveals that the laceration involves the eyelid margin medial to the right inferior punctum. *(continued)*

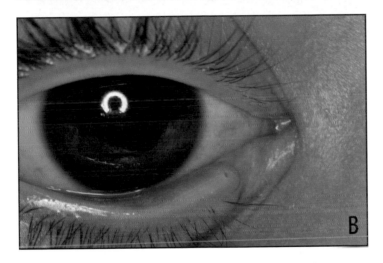

becoming adhered with glue. Positioning the patient so that the laceration is below the eye while applying the adhesive will prevent excess adhesive from flowing toward the eye from the wound. Despite this precaution, if the eyelids or lashes are accidentally glued together, the liberal application of a petrolatum-based ophthalmic ointment will allow the polymer to be gently dislodged in 24 hours.

Finally, in children, lacerations that are close to the eyelid margin or clearly through the margin are best inspected under general anesthesia and closed with sutures. First, it is difficult to approach the eye of an awake child without provoking a strong response, and it is even more difficult to prevent the adhesive from sticking to the lashes or from entering the palpebral aperture when applying it near the eyelid margin. More importantly, however, lacerations at the margin may involve the tarsal plate, the dense connective tissue in the posterior layer of the eyelid margin responsible for the support and shape of the lid. A laceration through the tarsus should not be closed with glue because the adhesive may not be strong enough to effect proper repair and because contracture of the tarsus at the eyelid margin could result in a "notch" or depression of the margin as it heals. This complication is best prevented with vertical mattress margin sutures. Further, in many cases, a laceration that at first appears to be a superficial scratch at the surface of the eyelid is in fact a deeper laceration involving the tarsal plate, and sometimes even the canaliculus if the wound is in the medial portion of the eyelid (Figure 16-1). Such lacerations are best explored under general anesthesia and sutured with absorbable sutures, taking care to intubate

Figure 16-1. (continued) (C) Probing the inferior punctum and canaliculus demonstrates a canalicular laceration; such an injury requires direct repair and stenting of the canaliculus, best performed under general anesthesia by a qualified ophthalmologist.

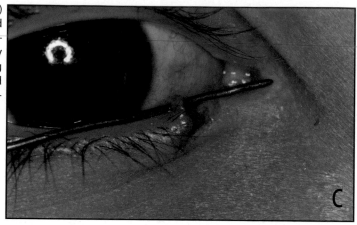

the canalicular ends or repair the tarsus as necessary. In cases of medial eyelid lacerations, the ophthalmologist passes a probe through the suspected lacerated canaliculus via the punctum and observes its course before attempting repair. All pediatric marginal eyelid lacerations with suspected canalicular involvement should be explored in the operating room within 48 hours to avoid potential canalicular scarring and permanent epiphora.

References

1. Mertz PM, Davis SC, Cazzaniga AL, Drosou A, Eaglstein WH. Barrier and antibacterial properties of 2-octyl cyanoacrylate-derived wound treatment films. *Journ Cutan Med Surg.* 2003;7(1):1-6.
2. Steiner Z, Mogliner J. Histoacryl vs dermabond cyanoacrylate glue for closing small operative wounds. *Harefuah.* 2000;139(11-12):409-411, 496.
3. Singer AJ, Hollander JE, Valentine SM, Turque TW, McCuskey CF, Quinn JV. Prospective, randomized, controlled trial of tissue adhesive (2-octylcyanoacrylate) vs standard wound closure techniques for laceration repair. Stony Brook Octylcyanoacrylate Study Group. *Acad Emerg Med.* 1998;5(2):94-99.
4. Singer AJ, Perry LC, Allen RL. In vivo study of wound bursting strength and compliance of topical skin adhesives. *Acad Emerg Med.* 2008;26(4):490-496.
5. Wackett, A, Singer AJ. The role of topical skin adhesives in wound repair. *Emer Med.* 2009;41(8):31-32, 34-35.

SECTION IV

INFECTIONS

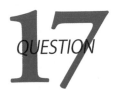
WHAT IS THE DIFFERENCE BETWEEN A STYE (HORDEOLUM) AND A CHALAZION, AND HOW ARE THEY TREATED?

Steven J. Lichtenstein, MD, FAAP

The phone rings in your office on Monday morning with a call from a mother who is in a panic. Her 2-year-old child has had a "bump" on her lower lid for approximately 3 days, but when she awoke this morning it was "bigger" and "redder," and she is really worried. You tell the mom to bring her baby in, and on examination you see a large red lesion on her right lower lid (Figure 17-1). There is no discharge, but the lesion does look like it is infected. What is the lesion, and what needs to be done to cure it? Is it an infection (a hordeolum or stye), or is it a blocked meibomian gland (a chalazion), and how is each one treated?

Clinical Characteristics

A *stye* or *hordeolum* is an infection of the perifollicular glands at the base of the eyelashes, also known as the glands of Moll and Zeiss (Figure 17-2). A *chalazion* is not an infection, but rather a blockage of a meibomian gland, a gland in the lid that produces the lipid layer of the tear film (Figure 17-3). Any inflammation of the eyelid margins can cause both hordeola and chalazia. For the practitioner, telling the difference between the 2 can be difficult.

Hordeola usually start at the lid margin and are tender or painful. They will enlarge with swelling and erythema, along with discomfort, over 2 to 3 days. They will often drain either externally to the skin surface or internally to the conjunctival surface, and spontaneously resolve. Although they represent a true infection of the perifollicular glands, they rarely need to be treated with antibiotics.

A chalazion will usually start as a solid nodule in the lid and may not actually involve the lid margin. Because it does not represent an infection, it does not require antibiotic therapy. Although

Wagner R. *Curbside Consultation in Pediatric Ophthalmology: 49 Clinical Questions* (pp 83-86)
© 2014 SLACK Incorporated

Figure 17-1. Acute hordeolum of the right lower lid.

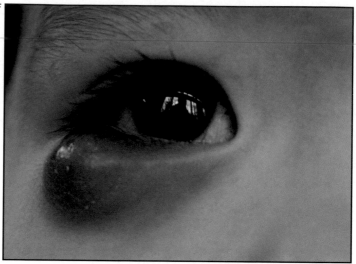

Figure 17-2. Anatomy of the lid showing perifollicular glands of Moll and Zeiss as well as meibomian glands.

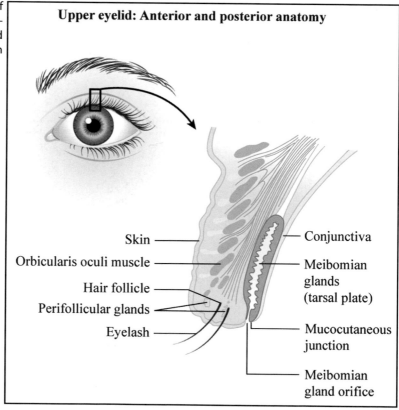

Upper eyelid: Anterior and posterior anatomy

Skin

Orbicularis oculi muscle

Hair follicle

Perifollicular glands

Eyelash

Conjunctiva

Meibomian glands (tarsal plate)

Mucocutaneous junction

Meibomian gland orifice

there might be mild tenderness associated with a chalazion, it will usually not be as tender as the hordeolum.

Because of the proximity of both the glands of Moll and Zeiss, as well as the meibomian glands to the lid margin, any condition that causes inflammation at the lid margin can precipitate the development of either a hordeolum or chalazion. This inflammation is often associated with blepharitis, with the causative organism being *Staphylococcus aureus*. The *S aureus* is not infecting

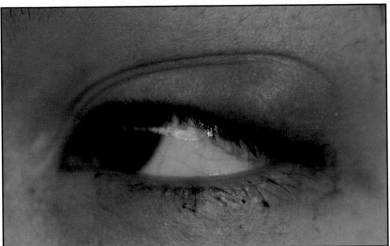

Figure 17-3. Chronic chalazion.

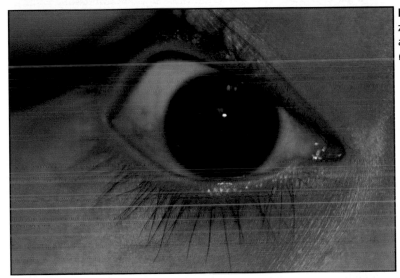

Figure 17-4. Chronic chalazion with staph blepharitis and conjunctival and corneal involvement.

the lid margin, but instead colonizing it at the base of the lashes and excreting an exotoxin to prevent other bacteria from colonizing the area. This inflammation is what needs to be addressed. Lid scrubs with diluted baby shampoo and antibiotics to the lash margin can help control the blepharitis. If the blepharitis becomes chronic, the *Staphylococcus aureus* exotoxin can cause corneal changes (Figure 17-4), with conjunctival injection and the corneal lesion noted at 8 o'clock at the limbus. These lesions can cause permanent corneal scarring if not addressed and treated.

Treatment

As mentioned previously, treatment of blepharitis, if it is present, is the primary concern to try to prevent recurrent episodes of hordeola and chalazia. Warm, moist compresses to the lid, started as quickly as possible, are the mainstay of therapy for both. Using a warm, wet washcloth for 10 to 15 minutes (or as long as the child will allow it) 3 to 6 times a day will speed resolution. Starting the warm compresses at the first appearance of the swelling and/or redness is the key to speedy resolution. Some parents have said that the washcloth will not stay warm (above body temperature) for any length of time, no matter how hot the water used to heat the cloth. One trick is to use a hardboiled egg or small potato as a "heat sink" inside of the wet washcloth. When a hardboiled egg with shell removed or a microwaved small potato is placed within the warm, wet washcloth, heat will be kept on the lid for a sustained period of time. The use of antibiotics either topically or systemically is not necessary, although the hordeolum represents a true infection of the perifollicular glands. With the use of the warm compresses, the lesions will usually drain and resolve without sequelae. If there is evidence of a true periorbital cellulitis, the use of oral antibiotics would be of benefit to treat the infection. However, this is a rare occurrence if the warm compresses are started as early as possible after the edema and erythema are noted.

In treating a chalazion, the use of an antibiotic is not indicated because these represent blockage of the meibomian glands and not an infectious process. If blepharitis is present, the use of a topical antibiotic to control the inflammation or to control meibomian gland dysfunction might be helpful in preventing recurrent episodes but is not as helpful as the warm compresses in the acute phase. If the child is a teenager, either tetracycline or doxycycline can be used to help emulsify the lipids that are being blocked in the clogged meibomian glands. But remember, the chalazion does not represent an infection. The judicious use of tetracycline or doxycycline in a child can cause significant discoloration of the permanent teeth and should be used with care and only in older children. If the child uses eye makeup she should be instructed to discontinue the use of all makeup until the lesion completely resolves and to discard any used products.

Because both chalazia and hordeola tend to be chronic in occurrence, control of lid margin disease is necessary in the long-term care of these children. If conservative acute treatment fails, surgical treatment might be necessary to resolve the problem and prevent permanent deformity to the lid.

Suggested Readings

Ellis FD. Chalazion. In: Wright KW, Spiegel PH, eds. *Pediatric Ophthalmol Strabismus*. 2nd ed. St Louis, MO: Mosby; 2003.

Holmstrom G. Hordeolum. In: Taylor D, Hoyt CS, eds. *Pediatric Ophthalmol Strabismus*. 3rd ed. Philadelphia, PA: Elsevier; 2005.

Hordeolum and chalazion. In: Gerstenblith AT, Rabinowitz MP, eds. *The Wills Eye Manual: Office and Emergency Room Diagnosis and Treatment of Eye Disorders*. 3rd ed. Philadelphia, PA: Lippincott Williams & Wilkins; 1999.

Iyengar S. The eyelids, chalazion. In: Olitsky SE, Nelson LB, eds. *A Color Handbook – Pediatric Clinical Ophthalmology*. London, England: Manson Publishing; 2012:190.

Iyengar S. The eyelids, hordeolum. In: Olitsky SE, Nelson LB, eds. *A Color Handbook–Pediatric Clinical Ophthalmology*. London, England: Manson Publishing; 2012:190.

HOW CAN I DETERMINE IF A RED EYE IS CAUSED BY A BACTERIAL INFECTION, VIRAL INFECTION, OR ALLERGIC REACTION? HOW ARE THEY MANAGED?

Christina M. Ohnsman, MD

In a patient presenting with a red eye, the primary concern is to rule out dangerous causes of redness, such as iritis or corneal abnormalities. Ask about pain, photophobia, loss of vision, history of injury, and contact lens use. If any of these warning signals are present, do a careful examination of the eye and consider an ophthalmic consult.

Assuming that this is a typical case of a red eye, or pink eye, the next step is to differentiate between infectious and allergic conjunctivitis. The history is a good starting place: Has the patient recently been exposed to peers with infectious conjunctivitis? Is there a history of environmental allergy? Are other symptoms of infection present, such as fever, pharyngitis, or earache, or are there allergy symptoms such as an itchy throat? Has there been any discharge? If so, have the patient or parent describe it. Is the eye itchy?

Your examination should include palpation for preauricular nodes, a sign of infectious conjunctivitis. Examine the eye for discharge, noting the quality and quantity. Infectious conjunctivitis may or may not be accompanied by a mucopurulent discharge (Figure 18-1), whereas allergic conjunctivitis is usually accompanied by tearing (Figure 18-2) and occasionally by a small amount of white, ropy, mucoid discharge. The presence of chemosis—conjunctival edema that looks like a raised bubble—is nearly pathognomonic for allergic conjunctivitis. Table 18-1 summarizes the findings that differentiate infectious from allergic conjunctivitis.

Allergic conjunctivitis is effectively treated with topical antihistamines and mast cell stabilizers, particularly those that do not sting upon instillation. Because children generally do not like eye drops, it is often wise to prescribe one that is given only once or twice a day. These drops may be used in combination with systemic antihistamines.

Distinguishing bacterial from viral conjunctivitis is a less straightforward process. Standard textbooks describe bacterial conjunctivitis as having bilateral onset of mucopurulent discharge,

Wagner R. *Curbside Consultation in Pediatric Ophthalmology: 49 Clinical Questions* (pp 87-89)
© 2014 SLACK Incorporated

Figure 18-1. Bacterial conjunctivitis with mucopurulent discharge.

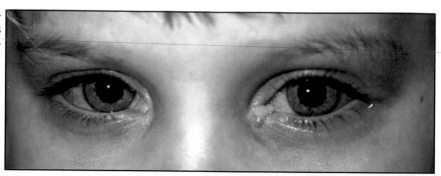

Figure 18-2. Red eye with watery discharge due to allergic conjunctivitis.

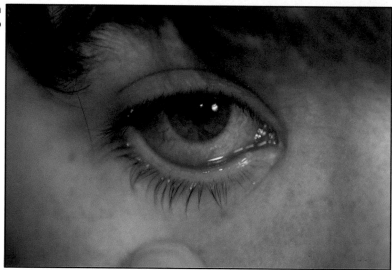

Table 18-1
Findings That Differentiate Infectious From Allergic Conjunctivitis

Infectious Conjunctivitis	*Allergic Conjunctivitis*
+/- mucopurulent discharge	+/- stringy or ropy mucous discharge
+/- tearing	Tearing
Unilateral or bilateral	Usually bilateral
No itching	Itching
No chemosis	+/- chemosis
+/- preauricular adenopathy	No adenopathy

occurring most commonly in preschoolers. On the other hand, the standard descriptions of viral conjunctivitis include unilateral onset of nonpurulent, watery discharge, accompanied by preauricular adenopathy, occurring most commonly in older children. We now know that this is not always the case. In 2002, an epidemic of infectious conjunctivitis at Princeton and Dartmouth Universities, and later in elementary schools in Maine, was caused by a novel strain of *Streptococcus pneumoniae*. These patients had variable findings, ranging from mildly inflamed conjunctiva with a clear, watery discharge to severe conjunctival inflammation with purulent discharge and preauricular adenopathy.[1] A number of other studies have confirmed that the presence or absence of discharge or preauricular adenopathy is not pathognomonic for bacterial or viral conjunctivitis.[2,3]

Given the above, how may we make treatment decisions in a given patient with infectious conjunctivitis? We do know that the presence of pharyngitis or gastroenteritis is suggestive of a viral etiology, particularly adenovirus, whereas otitis media suggests bacterial infection. Conjunctival cultures would not be practical due to the delay in receiving results. This leaves us with statistics: approximately 80% of the time, acute conjunctivitis in the pediatric population is due to bacterial infection.[4,5] For this reason, most cases of infectious conjunctivitis are treated with topical antibiotics, with fourth-generation fluoroquinolones being the treatment of choice. Older antibiotics, including previous-generation fluoroquinolones, are not recommended due to their limited spectrum of activity as well as high rates of resistance. In many cases, such as in the Ivy League outbreak, older antibiotics failed to decrease the duration of illness at all.[1] Addressing resistance concerns with fourth-generation fluoroquinolone use, a recent study showed that topical moxifloxacin in conjunctivitis did not lead to the development of resistant organisms in the eye or at distal body sites.[6]

In otitis-conjunctivitis syndrome, usually caused by *Haemophilus influenzae*, oral antibiotics are required. Likewise, in neonatal conjunctivitis, systemic antibiotic treatment is required. In cases that are highly suspicious for a viral etiology, no specific treatment is currently available. These patients may use warm or cool compresses for comfort and are often offered topical antibiotics in case they actually have bacterial conjunctivitis. All patients with infectious conjunctivitis are instructed to use strict measures to avoid contagion, including frequent hand-washing and exclusion from school until their symptoms resolve.

References

1. Centers for Disease Control and Prevention. Outbreak of bacterial conjunctivitis at a college: New Hampshire, January-March, 2002. *MMWR Morb Mortal Wkly Rep.* 2002;51:205-207.
2. Rietveld RP, vanWeert HCPM, ter Riet G, Bindels PJE. Diagnostic impact of signs and symptoms in acute infectious conjunctivitis: systematic literature search. *BMJ.* 2003;327:789.
3. Meltzer JA, Kunkov S, Crain EF. Identifying children at low risk for bacterial conjunctivitis. *Arch Pediatr Adolesc Med.* 2010;164(3):263-267.
4. Patel PB, Diaz MC, Bennett JE. Clinical features of bacterial conjunctivitis in children. *Acad Emerg Med.* 2007;14:1-5.
5. Weiss A, Brinser JH, Nazar-Stewart V. Acute conjunctivitis in childhood. *J Pediatr.* 1993;122:10-14.
6. Lichtenstein SJ, De Leon L, Heller W, et al. Topical ophthalmic moxifloxacin elicits minimal or no selection of fluoroquinolone resistance among bacteria isolated from the skin, nose, and throat. *J Pediatr Ophthalmol Strabismus.* 2012;49(2):88-97.

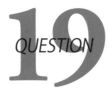

WHAT ARE THE SIGNS AND SYMPTOMS OF HERPES SIMPLEX IN THE EYE?

Jonathan C. Song, MD and Ismael Al Ghamdi, MD

Herpes simplex virus (HSV) keratitis is an important cause of ocular morbidity that can cause significant vision loss due to its recurring nature. It is caused by the same 2 closely related viruses: herpes simplex virus type 1 (HSV-1) and herpes simplex virus type 2 (HSV-2). HSV-1 is the first member of the human herpes viruses (HHV-1) belonging to the subfamily *Alphaherpesviridae*. At least 80% of the world's population has been exposed to HSV-1.

Children with HSV keratitis pose a unique challenge to the clinician. The most serious concern in children is that they are susceptible to amblyopia (lazy eye) from corneal scarring that may occur. The virus is transmitted from human to human via secreted fluids and close contact with mucosal surfaces or abraded skin. Initial infection is usually asymptomatic and occurs in children younger than 5 years old. In cases of HSV-2, it is transmitted as the newborn passes through an infected birth canal. Ocular infection may occur directly through droplet spread or indirectly via neuronal spread from a nonocular site such as the oral mucosa.

HSV keratitis occurs when the infection reaches the corneal epithelium and stroma of the cornea. Manifestations can include cutaneous vesicles, blepharitis, conjunctivitis, epithelial keratitis (corneal dendritic ulcers), and stromal keratitis. Nonspecific signs of primary herpetic corneal infection include fever, malaise, and lymphadenopathy. When the virus gains access to the central nervous system, the virus becomes latent in the trigeminal ganglia (HSV-1 or varicella–zoster virus [VZV]) or in the spinal ganglia (HSV-2). Recurrent attacks occur when the virus travels peripherally via sensory nerves to infect target tissues in the eye. These attacks may be triggered by any of the following stressors: fever, ultraviolet light exposure, trauma, stress, menses, and immunosuppression.

Recurrent ocular HSV-1 infection and inflammation eventually cause corneal scarring, thinning, neovascularization, and stromal keratitis. This disease usually occurs unilaterally, but

Wagner R. *Curbside Consultation in Pediatric Ophthalmology: 49 Clinical Questions* (pp 91-92) © 2014 SLACK Incorporated

Figure 19-1. Herpes simplex dendrite on cornea seen with fluorescein staining and blue light.

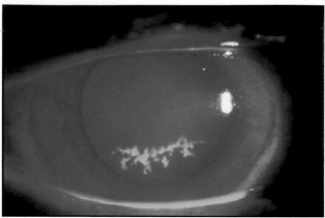

bilateral infection, although not frequently seen, usually afflicts a younger age group and can be more severe. The corneal dendrites of herpes simplex infections are epithelial ulcers whose edges stain brightly with fluorescein and have terminal bulbs (Figure 19-1). Herpes zoster dendrites are raised lesions, do not have terminal bulbs, and do not stain well with fluorescein. Some ophthalmic findings of HSV keratitis are not directly caused by the viral infection itself, but instead relate to the immunologic response to the infection, such as chronic keratouveitis (inflammation within the anterior chamber of the eye) and disciform and necrotizing keratitis (cornea is filled with inflammatory cells and has neovascularization despite an intact surface).

HSV keratitis in children may differ from that in adults. The rate of bilateral involvement in the largest series of infected children was 10% to 26%, which is higher than seen in adults. The Herpetic Eye Disease Study estimated that both epithelial and stromal keratitis recurred in 18% of patients during a follow-up period of 18 months. Age, sex, ethnicity, and nonocular herpes were not significantly associated with recurrences. However, the Herpetic Eye Disease Study was limited to patients 12 years or older. In different series of pediatric herpetic viral keratitis, recurrence rates ranged from 33% to 80%. Corneal scarring and ulcerations from recurrent herpetic keratitis can be visually debilitating and potentially necessitate surgical intervention with penetrating keratoplasty (corneal transplantation) or tarsorrhaphy (partial lid closure). The inflammatory response from herpetic keratitis leads to stromal scarring and opacification and tends to be more severe in children than adults. For younger children, especially under age 8, the corneal opacity and irregular astigmatism induced by the scars lead to visual deprivation and loss of vision. Even with antiviral therapy, corneal healing can take up to 1 month and will require continued ophthalmic care due to residual corneal scarring and risk of vision loss.

Suggested Readings

Hsiao CH, Yeung L, Yeh LK, et al. Pediatric herpes simplex virus keratitis. *Cornea*. 2004;28(3):249-253.

Stanberry LR. *Understanding Herpes*. Jackson, MS: University Press of Mississippi; 2006.

Toma HS, Murina AT, Areaux RG, et al. Ocular HSV-1 latency, reactivation, and recurrent disease. *Semin Ophthalmol*. 2008;23:249-273.

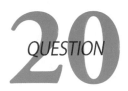

IS IT EVER APPROPRIATE FOR A NON-OPHTHALMOLOGIST PHYSICIAN TO USE TOPICAL STEROIDS FOR OCULAR DISEASE?

Kara Cavuoto, MD and Mark Dorfman, MD

Due to the frequency of children with a red eye presenting to the clinic and the common inflammatory pathophysiology between many of the inciting causes, some primary care providers have developed a comfort level in prescribing topical steroids. This may be in the form of an ophthalmic drop, ocular ointment, or periocular cream. Subsequently, we see children presenting to our pediatric ophthalmology clinic who have been unsuccessfully treated with steroid-containing drops such as dexamethasone/tobramycin (Tobradex) for diagnoses such as chalazia or atopic conjunctivitis. However, the authors advise pediatricians not to write a prescription for an ocular steroid given the potential for exposing the child to a permanent visual impairment if the appropriate diagnosis is not made.

Steroids are anti-inflammatory agents that have uses in nearly every realm of medicine. As synthetic glucocorticoids, they induce changes in the body that are similar to the naturally occurring hormone cortisol. They act to prevent or suppress inflammation at the cellular, tissue, and biochemical levels. Within the realm of ophthalmology, they can be applied topically to the eyelids or to the globe, injected subconjunctivally or intravitreally, or orally dosed.

There are many different commercially available steroid-containing drops and ointments, as well as combined steroid-antibiotic agents. Table 20-1 details some of the more commonly used preparations. The dosing recommendations usually start at 4 times daily, depending on the severity of the inflammation.

When prescribed appropriately, topical steroids are effective and play a role in treating ophthalmic pathology. Common conditions ophthalmologists treat with steroids include allergic or vernal conjunctivitis, uveitis, blepharitis, hypersensitivity ulcers secondary to *Staphylococcus*, chalazia, postoperative states, and severe atopic dermatitis (Table 20-2).

Wagner R. *Curbside Consultation in Pediatric
Ophthalmology: 49 Clinical Questions* (pp 93-97)
© 2014 SLACK Incorporated

Table 20-1

Commonly Used Steroid-Only and Steroid-Antibiotic Medications

Commonly Used Steroid-Only Medications

Generic Name	Trade Name	Preparation
Fluorometholone 0.1%	FML 0.1%	Suspension, ointment
Loteprednol 0.5%	Lotemax	Suspension
Loteprednol 0.2%	Alrex	Suspension
Difluprednate 0.05%	Durezol	Suspension
Prednisolone 1%	PredForte, OmniPred	Suspension
Prednisolone 0.1%	PredMild	Suspension

Commonly Used Steroid-Antibiotic Medications

Generic Name	Trade Name	Preparation
Dexamethasone/neomycin sulfate/polymyxin B sulfate	Maxitrol	Suspension, ointment
Dexamethasone/tobramycin	Tobradex	Suspension, ointment
Prednisolone acetate/sulfacetamide	Blephamide	Suspension, ointment

Table 20-2

Uses for Topical Steroids by Ophthalmologists

Indication

- Allergic or vernal conjunctivitis
- Uveitis
- Blepharitis
- Hypersensitivity ulcers secondary to *Staphylococcus*
- Chalazia
- Postoperative states
- Atopic dermatitis

Children presenting with itching, redness, and thick whitish discharge predominantly in the spring or summer months are often diagnosed with *allergic conjunctivitis*. Most cases of atopic conjunctivitis can be treated with topical mast cell stabilizers/antihistamine drops. However, a more severe form of allergic conjunctivitis is *vernal conjunctivitis*. Topical steroids are necessary to treat the significant inflammation that is present. Because treatment may be necessary for a longer period of time, steroids with lower strength and fewer side effects will be used, such as fluorometholone or loteprednol.

Uveitis, particularly anterior uveitis, is typically an idiopathic and noninfectious inflammation that presents with redness, pain, photophobia, and decreased vision in the affected eye. However, anterior uveitis in juvenile idiopathic arthritis will present with no symptoms. It should be noted that recurrent and/or bilateral cases warrant a systemic evaluation because they may be associated with autoimmune conditions, such as juvenile idiopathic arthritis, or infectious conditions such as tuberculosis, syphilis or toxoplasmosis. The treatment of uveitis requires a stronger steroid, such as prednisolone acetate 1%, as frequently as every hour upon treatment initiation.

Blepharitis is a bilateral inflammation of the eyelid margin associated with itching, burning, tearing, and crusting around the eyelids. Other common findings include red, thickened eyelid margins with inspissated oil glands. Treatment regimens include scrubbing the eyelid margins with mild shampoo, warm compresses, preservative-free artificial tears, and, for more severe cases, a topical steroid-containing ointment. Blepharitis can be associated with *phlyctenulosis* (small white nodules on the conjunctiva or cornea), and *Staphylococcus* marginal disease (multiple small white corneal opacities), due to a delayed hypersensitivity to the *Staphylococcus* present on the eyelid margin

A *chalazion* is a focal area of inflammation surrounding an obstructed meibomian gland. This often presents as a visible, well-defined subcutaneous nodule in the upper or lower eyelid of one or both eyes. Treatment includes warm compresses 4 times daily, lid hygiene to treat concurrent blepharitis, and a steroid-containing drop or ointment 4 times daily. Occasionally, the chalazion may fail to resolve with conservative treatment, and surgical incision and drainage may be required.

A primary infection with herpes simplex virus (HSV) is associated with a unilateral or bilateral "red eye" with pain, photophobia, decreased vision, and a vesicular skin rash. Recurrent HSV infections present with unilateral redness, pain, and frequently no vesicular rash. This may make these reactivations or recurrences difficult to distinguish from other forms of conjunctivitis. The only diagnostic sign is dendritic keratitis, which may be found on a slit lamp examination. Severe cases may result in stromal melting and corneal perforation. Acute treatment will be decided by the presentation of the keratitis but usually includes oral acyclovir. Once the keratitis has become inactive and healed, a corneal scar forms and results in blurred vision, irregular astigmatism, and amblyopia. The ophthalmologist may use steroids to treat the significant inflammation associated with herpetic infections, but this is done in combination with topical antiviral agents such as Viroptic (trifluridine).

Postoperative implementation of steroids is used to decrease the inflammatory reaction to the surgical event. This is especially common in children who have had strabismus surgery, cataract extraction, and retinal surgery. We often recommend the parents apply an antibiotic-steroid combination drop or ointment, such as Maxitrol or Tobradex (tobramycin and dexamethasone ophthalmic), to the ocular surface 4 times daily for the first 5 days after surgery. This is often sufficient to prevent infection and decrease the expected postoperative inflammation.

Even with the numerous beneficial uses, steroids should be prescribed with careful attention to the potential side effects and ocular sequelae (Table 20-3). We strongly recommend that physicians who cannot examine the integrity of the corneal epithelium with the benefit of a slit lamp should not prescribe topical steroids. If steroids are prescribed without a thorough examination of the cornea, primary care physicians place their patients in danger of sight-threatening complications

Table 20-3

Dangers and Side Effects of Topical Steroids

Danger	Ophthalmologic Manifestations
Glaucoma	Elevated intraocular pressure
	Damage to optic nerve
	Loss of peripheral visual field
Cataracts	Decreased central visual acuity
	Amblyopia from visual deprivation
	Postcataract extraction complications (endophthalmitis, glaucoma)
Depression of immune system	Worsening of existing infection
	Herpetic keratitis
	Corneal ulcers
	Fungal infections
	Acanthamoeba
	Scarring of the central visual axis (deprivation amblyopia)

with lifelong sequelae. This is especially true in the pediatric population where the child may not be able to voice or localize decreased vision, increased pain, or photophobia.

The most severe complication of indiscriminate steroid use is opacification of the central visual axis due to scarring. This is particularly devastating to a child because the permanent scar causes visual deprivation and thus irreversible amblyopia. These opacities cannot be treated with corneal transplantation due to the low success rate in the pediatric population. Two common disease processes that are associated with residual corneal scars are herpetic keratitis and corneal ulcers.

Beyond potentiating herpetic keratitis, the presence of a steroid enables bacteria, fungi, and parasites such as *Acanthamoeba* to proliferate and destroy the cornea. This occurs because steroids compromise the immune system and prevent normal corneal healing. Primary care providers must take particular precautions in children with a red eye who wear contact lenses. Bacterial ulcers can result from wearing contact lenses for extended hours, as well as microabrasions from insertion and removal of the lens.

Cataracts, especially the posterior subcapsular type, have a strong association with chronic steroid use. The presence of the cataract causes a gradual decrease in visual acuity and creates amblyopia from visual deprivation. A cataract may be surgically extracted; however, this also places the child at risk for subsequent complications associated with intraocular surgery, including endophthalmitis and glaucoma.

Other than the amblyogenic outcomes of corneal scars and cataracts, numerous other side effects result from imprudent steroid use. Steroids result in elevation of the intraocular pressure and the development of glaucoma, which may have no noticeable signs outside of the ophthalmic examination. Intraocular pressure is difficult to measure in an awake child and is often unreliable if checked in the clinic due to limited cooperation. In addition, the child may not recognize or not be able to vocalize the loss of the peripheral visual field. Due to this combination of factors, the diagnosis is often delayed and irreversible loss of the peripheral visual field has already occurred.

Parents tend to keep topical drops after treatment and will frequently pull these drops out to treat a red eye that may occur weeks or months later. It is imperative that when topical steroids are prescribed, the family is warned to discard the bottle after the treatment regimen. The chronic use of steroids in this manner will result in one of the side effects listed previously and likely lead to a permanent and irreversible loss of vision. Furthermore, the pediatrician should also recognize that a prescription for a steroid should never be written with unlimited refills or refilled without knowing the status of the condition being treated by the steroid. These drops can safely be renewed as long as there has been a comprehensive evaluation by the pediatric ophthalmologist.

Conclusion

Topical steroids should not be used without a slit lamp evaluation and an assessment of intraocular pressure. There are times that topical steroids are necessary, and the primary care provider needs to consult with the ophthalmologist to avoid unnecessary complications with sight-threatening side effects.

Suggested Readings

Baratz KH, Hattenhauer MG. Indiscriminate use of corticosteroid-containing eyedrops. *Mayo Clin Proc.* 1999;74(4):362-366.

Hutcheson KA. Steroid-induced glaucoma in an infant. *J AAPOS.* 2007;11(5):522-523.

Lam DS, Fan DS, Ng JS, Yu CB, Wong CY, Cheung AY. Ocular hypertensive and anti-inflammatory responses to different dosages of topical dexamethasone in children: a randomized trial. *Clin Experiment Ophthalmol.* 2005;33(3):252-258.

How Do I Know When to Admit a Child With Orbital Cellulitis to the Hospital?

Dorothy J. Reynolds, MD

A child presents for evaluation of eyelid swelling and erythema. At first glance, this may appear to be an obvious or simple problem; however, hidden behind the swollen lids can be signs of a potentially vision- or life-threatening condition. To make the proper diagnosis, critical considerations include patient age, clinical findings of infection, and the extent of the disease process, whether *preseptal* or *orbital*. Preseptal cellulitis may evolve into orbital cellulitis, and treatment needs to be appropriately aggressive, while orbital cellulitis may be complicated by vision loss, abscess formation, or spread to the brain. History and examination will guide you, and at times imaging is helpful or required.

Throughout evaluation of such a patient, I continuously think in terms of the extent of the infection, whether preseptal or orbital (not periorbital, which essentially means "around the eye"). This differentiation depends on the infection location in relation to the orbital septum—a fibrous, multilayered connective tissue membrane arising from the periosteum of the superior and inferior orbital rims, fusing in the anterior eyelids with the levator aponeurosis superiorly and the tarsus inferiorly. The orbital septum delineates the anterior superficial tissues and skin of the eyelid and adjacent face (preseptal) from the deeper posterior structures of the orbit and globe (orbital). The septum is not an absolute barrier, and infection may indeed spread through it.

You cannot externally visualize the septum; however, severity of disease and clinical findings generally vary based on infection location in relation to this structure. Preseptal cellulitis is a more superficial infection involving the eyelid and soft tissue anterior to the septum, without extension to the deeper orbital structures. Orbital cellulitis is a more serious infection of the deeper postseptal structures. Preseptal findings include eyelid swelling and erythema with possible tenderness, an essentially quiet eye (maybe minimal injection), and possibly mild fever. Findings of orbital cellulitis include those of preseptal cellulitis plus any of the following: pain, ophthalmoplegia, pain with eye movement, eye redness/congestion, globe proptosis/displacement or resistance to retropulsion, abnormal pupillary reaction, decreased vision, retinal venous congestion, or optic nerve edema. To differentiate preseptal from orbital cellulitis you must evaluate the eye and its

Wagner R. *Curbside Consultation in Pediatric*
Ophthalmology: 49 Clinical Questions (pp 99-102)
© 2014 SLACK Incorporated

function and consider severity of signs and symptoms (this disease spectrum can and does evolve). If there is any suggestion of an orbital process, you must consider further investigation with imaging.

Preseptal cellulitis may result from skin trauma of the lid/brow/face, allowing organism entry (eg, insect bite, laceration/puncture/wound), upper respiratory infection or sinusitis, adjacent infection (eg, conjunctivitis, dacryocystitis, impetigo), or infected hordeolum. When there is no evident skin source (most common etiology), preseptal cellulitis is generally secondary to sinusitis. Orbital cellulitis is a more serious infection that may evolve from preseptal cellulitis (perhaps inadequately treated) but is most often secondary to sinusitis, especially ethmoiditis. Orbital cellulitis may also develop from adjacent infection (eg, dacryocystitis, infection of the eye or extraocular muscles); eyelid/orbital trauma, including complication of orbital fracture or retained foreign body; complication of periorbital/eye/sinus surgery; or hematogenous or bacteremic spread (eg, dental infection/abscess, otitis media).

History

As always, the history can be revealing. While focusing on the present disease and its course, your aim is to identify the source and extent of the infection and reveal systemic signs suggestive of a sicker child. Key points to consider include recent wound/trauma (eye, orbit, nearby face), infection (eye, sinus, upper respiratory, ear, dental), and surgery (eye, orbit, sinus, face, dental). Prior episodes and treatment are relevant to identifying a recurrent or chronic process. Medical history must be reviewed for immunosuppression, cancer, diabetes mellitus (increased risk for mucormycosis), upper respiratory infection, and sinusitis. Ocular history is important, including prior surgery, recent injury, or infection. Review of systems should include pain, fever, vomiting, headache, mental status changes, meningeal symptoms, and lethargy.

Clinical Examination

On clinical examination, general concerns include vital signs, mental status, and constitutional signs of infection, especially of the upper respiratory system and sinuses (eg, nasal discharge, sinus congestion). Look for evidence of periorbital and adjacent facial skin trauma, and if a wound is present, explore it. Inspect the eyelids, noting location and degree of swelling, redness, warmth, and tenderness, as well as any discharge. Feel for a fluctuant mass (possible abscess).

Thoroughly examine the eyes by inspecting the globe and checking the vision, ocular motility, and pupils. These steps are critical to a clinical determination of the extent of infection, whether preseptal or orbital. I need to stress that if a complete eye examination cannot be performed or you are concerned by any findings, it is absolutely reasonable and indeed necessary to promptly consult an ophthalmologist. If the lids are swollen shut, with no unaided view of the eye, you will need to manually separate them (lift the skin over the orbital rim). If there is severe lid swelling and tenderness, this may require reassurance and probably parental help by holding the child in a hug, followed by prying open the lids as best you can. If you are met with considerable resistance and/or there is a recent history of trauma to or around the eye, it is prudent to maintain concern for a serious eye injury, including possible globe trauma and/or retained foreign body, and defer further urgent evaluation to an ophthalmologist. Otherwise, inspect the globe for signs of trauma, infection, conjunctival injection/chemosis, and discharge. Check the monocular vision in each eye. Assess for a pupillary abnormality (afferent pupillary defect). Evaluate the ocular motility for 360 degrees, comparing the position of each eye to highlight a deficit, and assess for pain with eye movement. Inspect for globe displacement (the corneal light reflex should be aligned symmetrically in both eyes) and proptosis (look from above at a bird's-eye view for protrusion of the eye). Assess for resistance to globe retropulsion. An ophthalmologist will also evaluate the retina for venous congestion and optic nerve edema.

A diagnosis of preseptal cellulitis is suggested by eyelid erythema and swelling, with possible tenderness. There is a quiet eye (perhaps mild conjunctival injection but no chemosis/bogginess), no pain, no limitation of ocular motility, no pain with eye movement, no globe proptosis/displacement or resistance to retropulsion, normal vision and pupils, and possibly mild fever. The child is generally less sick (though this can be deceiving). Orbital cellulitis is instead suggested by findings of preseptal cellulitis plus any of the following: limitation of ocular motility, pain (possibly worse with eye movement), double vision, globe proptosis/displacement or resistance to retropulsion, globe injection or chemosis, decreased periorbital sensation, decreased vision, abnormal pupillary reflex, retinal venous congestion, or optic nerve edema. Remember that this is a disease spectrum, and clinically apparent moderate to severe preseptal cellulitis may in fact be early orbital cellulitis. Also, headache, fever, mental status changes, meningeal signs, or lethargy may indicate a sicker and even toxic child; do not forget this process can spread to the brain. Imaging may ultimately be necessary to make your diagnosis, clarify the extent of disease, and assess for any complications.

Treatment

Treatment decisions depend on the severity and extent of infection, patient age, patient compliance, and whether the patient has failed systemic antibiotic therapy (worsening or no improvement). Mild preseptal cellulitis may generally be treated on an outpatient basis with broad-spectrum oral antibiotics for at least 10 days, daily follow-up until clearly improving, then close follow-up until completely resolved. Hospital admission and intravenous antibiotics are indicated when your patient has moderate to severe preseptal cellulitis, preseptal cellulitis that has worsened or not improved on systemic antibiotics, orbital cellulitis, and/or toxic signs or symptoms. In these cases, I recommend that you act fast, seriously consider imaging, and treat aggressively. The ultimate goal is to prevent progression of the disease or potential sight- and life-threatening complications, including orbital and subperiosteal abscess, cavernous sinus thrombosis, and/or intracranial infection, that require prolonged treatment and sometimes surgery (orbital, sinus, and/or neurosurgery).

There are additional caveats when considering patient admission, need for imaging, and treatment. First, any concern regarding compliance warrants admission. Next, the younger the child, the lower my threshold for patient admission, intravenous antibiotics, and possibly imaging. Some recommend admission for any child up to the age of 5 years, even for milder preseptal cellulitis. These younger children may be more challenging to evaluate, thereby escaping detection of early nuances of an orbital process, and they may progress more rapidly (thinner orbital septum thus a less effective barrier), thereby supporting earlier, more aggressive intervention. Next, any child with a limited examination requires urgent ophthalmology evaluation, as well as serious consideration for admission and/or imaging. Finally, there are some children who are worrisome and simply don't "feel" right based on your findings, despite falling outside the above guidelines. These children may have disease in transition, rapidly progressing infection, or early orbital signs that are clinically less apparent. In such a situation, ophthalmology evaluation and imaging are prudent, and admission for closer monitoring and/or intravenous antibiotics may be warranted to stave off disease progression.

All admitted patients need ophthalmology consultation and probable imaging. Computed tomography (CT) of the sinuses/orbits (and sometimes brain) is generally performed for patients in whom there is no external source of infection, limited examination, a diagnosis of orbital cellulitis, history of trauma, or concern for abscess or intracranial infection. Patients with moderate to severe preseptal cellulitis may also warrant imaging for the same reasons, or if they have failed oral antibiotics. Despite concern for radiation exposure, CT is superior to magnetic resonance imaging, and remains the imaging study of choice for these patients. CT should be obtained with and preferably also without contrast, including axial and coronal thin cuts, to elucidate the presence of sinusitis, orbital disease, orbital or subperiosteal abscess, cavernous sinus thrombosis, intracranial involvement, or retained foreign body.

On admission, obtain gram stain/culture/sensitivity of any eye/wound/nasal discharge/drainage, complete blood count with differential, and blood cultures with sensitivity. Broad-spectrum intravenous antibiotics must be promptly started. Decisions regarding antibiotic choice are patient dependent, and specific recommendations frequently change. I frequently advocate Pediatric Infectious Disease input regarding antibiotic regimen, as well as information on prevalent organisms in the community, keeping in mind the increasing occurrence of multidrug-resistant bacteria. Antibiotics may need to be broadened pending the patient's clinical response. Generally, intravenous antibiotics are maintained for at least 72 hours. At that point, if there is significant clinical improvement and the child is afebrile with known culture results, appropriate culture-directed oral antibiotics may be considered to complete a full 2-week course. Early ophthalmology involvement on admission will allow a baseline from which to monitor the patient's treatment response, which is critical to subsequent decisions for more aggressive treatment or the need for surgery. If the patient has sinusitis, this is generally the nidus of infection, and otolaryngology should be immediately consulted and nasal decongestant sprays promptly initiated. All patients with preseptal or orbital cellulitis also benefit from warm moist compresses to the lids if tolerated and topical antibiotics if any associated conjunctivitis.

Admitted children require meticulous follow-up, initially at least daily, dictated by the disease severity and response to treatment. Close follow-up is maintained until complete resolution. Inpatient stay may range from a few days to even weeks. Culture results and white blood cell count must be followed. Continuing headache or fever, clinical worsening or lack of improvement, worsening leukocytosis, and/or new findings despite intravenous antibiotics are worrisome for disease evolution or spread with complications that may warrant repeat imaging and/or more aggressive treatment, including additional antibiotic coverage or surgical intervention.

I encourage you to maintain a high index of suspicion throughout your evaluation and management of these patients. Proper diagnosis, early intervention, and appropriately aggressive treatment are key factors to help prevent disease progression and avoid serious complications. It is always better to err on the conservative side, whether hospital admission for closer monitoring, intravenous antibiotics, imaging to clarify the extent of disease, and/or earlier involvement of an ophthalmologist.

Suggested Readings

Bedwell J, Bauman N. Management of pediatric orbital cellulitis and abscess. *Curr Opin Otolaryngol Head Neck Surg.* 2011;19(6):467-473.

Ehlers JP, Shah CP, eds. *The Wills Eye Manual: Office and Emergency Room Diagnosis and Treatment of Eye Disease.* 5th ed. Philadelphia, PA: Lippincott Williams & Wilkins; 2008.

Hauser A, Fogarasi S. Periorbital and orbital cellulitis. *Pediatrics in Review.* 2010;31(6):242-249.

Reynolds DJ, Kodsi SR, Rubin SE, Rodgers IR. Intracranial infection associated with preseptal and orbital cellulitis in the pediatric patient. *J AAPOS.* 2003;7(6):413-417.

Rudloe TF, Harper MB, Prabhu SP, Rahbar R, VanderVeen D, Kimia AA. Acute periorbital infections: who needs emergent imaging? *Pediatrics.* 2010;125(4):719-726.

DOES MRSA CAUSE OCULAR DISEASE?

Rudolph S. Wagner, MD

There is no question that methicillin-resistant *Staphylococcus aureus* (MRSA) as a cause of ocular and orbital disease in children is on the rise. MRSA is most frequently involved in isolated cases of periocular skin and nasolacrimal duct infections and in a particular type of orbital cellulitis.

MRSA has been found to cause potentially serious and vision-threatening ocular disease including orbital cellulitis, dacrocystitis, keratitis, and endophthalmitis, with blepharoconjunctivitis representing 78% of MRSA ocular infections. The incidence of methicillin resistance in *S aureus* infections is on the rise in the United States, with one study showing an increase from 4.1% of ocular isolates in 1998 to 1999 to 16.7% in 2005 to 2006. MRSA was previously typically found in hospital settings, but the incidence of community-acquired MRSA (CA-MRSA) has been increasing, whereas the numbers of nosocomial infections has remained stable. Despite widespread fear of MRSA infection, symptoms have been found to be milder than expected, with few resulting in ocular morbidity and visual losses. At the present time, pediatric conjunctivitis caused by CA-MRSA has not been a problem, although individual case reports are surfacing. There have been a number of reports of orbital cellulitis in nonimmunocompromised children caused by MRSA. In most reports of MRSA ocular disease, strains have been sensitive to non-beta-lactam antibiotics such as vancomycin, trimethoprim, or topical mupirocin.

Wagner R. *Curbside Consultation in Pediatric
Ophthalmology: 49 Clinical Questions* (pp 103-107)
© 2014 SLACK Incorporated

MRSA Orbital Cellulitis in Contrast to Typical Bacterial Orbital Cellulitis

Orbital cellulitis caused by MRSA may result vision loss. Often, there may be a delay in diagnosis and referral for surgical intervention as a result of an atypical presentation in children. In fact, a recent study found that patients with MRSA-related orbital cellulitis had clinical and radiographic features typically not seen in cases of orbital cellulitis in children. In this series, there was development of eyelid swelling in the absence of a preceding upper respiratory illness or a traumatic skin injury. In contrast to usual cases of orbital cellulitis, only a small percentage of patients were found to have adjacent paranasal sinusitis, specifically only 17% in the pediatric population. There was also a high percentage of lacrimal gland abscesses in the pediatric subgroup. It is important to keep in mind that lid swelling in the absence of recent upper respiratory illness and the finding of a lacrimal gland focus of infection in a child are suggestive of MRSA orbital cellulitis. Perhaps more significantly, the clinical finding of multiple orbital abscesses and the absence of adjacent paranasal sinus disease are considered predictive factors suggestive of MRSA as the cause of orbital cellulitis. In children with the clinical picture described here, aggressive treatment for MRSA orbital cellulitis with empiric antibiotic coverage should be instituted. Immediate surgical drainage of any focal abscess should be considered as well.

The Neonatal Intensive Care Unit and MRSA Ocular Infections

Neonates are considered to be more susceptible to infections due to their immature immune systems. Therefore, physicians are tempted to empirically treat with broad-spectrum antibiotics to protect against pathogens such as MRSA. This perception is compounded by the practice of many neonatal intensive care units (NICU) to routinely culture all infants in their units at multiple sites of potential infection for MRSA. Despite many positive cultures, few babies are found to have MRSA-related disease. In particular, MRSA-related conjunctivitis is believed to occur infrequently in the NICU. Reported data indicate that it is often not necessary to treat conjunctivitis empirically for MRSA except if the patient possesses risk factors for infection. In one study analyzing hospital-acquired conjunctivitis in the NICU, 25% of cases were caused by coagulase-negative *Staphylococcus*, whereas 19% were due to *S aureus*. This study did not distinguish infection caused specifically by MRSA, but other investigations found that 73% of the *S aureus* isolates were MRSA. Clinically identified conjunctivitis was found to be associated with low birth weight and conditions that increased the risk of ocular contamination by respirator secretions, such as suctioning when on ventilators or continuous positive airway pressure and ocular examinations. In addition, the study investigated only hospital-acquired conjunctivitis in NICU patients, not community-acquired cases. Therefore, it would be expected that if the prevalence of MRSA was so low in a hospital setting, its presence in the community would be even less significant. Nevertheless, adherence to strict infection control procedures by health care workers as well as protective measures, such as eye protection, during suction may decrease the incidence of such disease.

A documented case of MRSA infection is illustrated in a 12-day-old infant who developed dacrocystitis and periorbital cellulitis. The mother was infected with a groin abscess during the first trimester of pregnancy and was successfully treated with clindamycin. The infant's blood cultures were identical to the organisms in the abscess, and therefore it was considered to be community acquired. The patient was likely colonized during vaginal delivery or contact shortly after birth

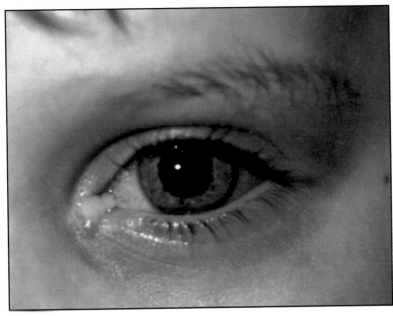

Figure 22-1. MRSA may present as a typical bacterial conjunctivitis with eyelid edema, conjunctival vascular injection, and a mucopurulent discharge as seen here.

but also had a nasolacrimal duct obstruction that promoted progression to infection. The neonate received intravenous vancomycin and topical polymyxin-trimethoprim ophthalmic solution, with rifampin initiated when the infant developed disseminated disease. The patient improved with treatment and was symptom free in 2 weeks.

CA-MRSA Conjunctivitis: Is It a Problem?

CA-MRSA conjunctivitis in children has been reported to occur with increased frequency in northern California. Many of these cases occurred in neonates and none were associated with significant ocular morbidity. MRSA conjunctivitis is also being diagnosed more frequently in adults. Patients who are infected by MRSA tend to present with conjunctivitis or blepharitis and may have a recurrence of infection, perhaps related to treatment with an ineffective topical antibiotic. Presently, infection with MRSA is not a significant concern in producing serious ocular disease in patients with conjunctivitis. Children infected with MRSA may present as a typical bacterial conjunctivitis with eyelid edema, conjunctival vascular injection, and mucopurulent discharge. In a child, these signs and symptoms may be indistinguishable from the typical bacterial conjunctivitis caused by *Streptococcus pneumonia* and *Haemophilus influenzae* (Figure 22-1). A diagnostic clue might be a failure of the conjunctivitis to respond to a topical antibiotic such as an aminoglycoside. MRSA conjunctivitis occurring in an immunocompromised child might result in significant morbidity if left untreated.

Atypical cases of necrotizing CA-MRSA causing palpebral conjunctival ulceration, destruction of postseptal soft tissue, and invasion of extraconal fat have been reported in immunocompetent individuals. Such severe cases are rare, and physicians should consider MRSA infection and treat accordingly if such atypical necrotizing, invading conjunctivitis develops. Appropriate empirical treatment is vancomycin until culture sensitivities narrow therapy. Surgical intervention may be necessary if infection progresses to abscess formation that is resistant to antibiotic penetration. Adults also usually carry additional risk factors that predispose them to ocular infection by

MRSA. These risks are greatest in health care workers, athletes with close physical contact; and immunocompromised patients such as those with diabetes mellitus, those taking steroids, and those postsurgery, especially cataract removal and LASIK.

Treatment of MRSA Ocular Infections

When children present with significant orbital and ocular disease caused by or suspected to be caused by MRSA, systemic antibiotics such as trimethoprim and vancomycin are available and effective. Unfortunately for cases of conjunctivitis caused by or suspected to be caused by MRSA, topical vancomycin is not available commercially and requires compounding by a pharmacist to prepare drops for ocular instillation. The commercially available topical combination of polymyxin B and trimethoprim sulfate as well as topical gentamycin may be effective in cases of conjunctivitis caused by MRSA. Although a MRSA isolate may be classified as resistant to fluoroquinolones, such high concentrations of antibiotic are delivered topically to the site of the infection that the minimum inhibitory concentration (MIC) is greatly exceeded, and the antibiotic may be effective even if the specific organism's MIC would technically classify the organism as resistant. Most cases of MRSA conjunctivitis are resistant to erythromycin.

Given the low prevalence and incidence of MRSA among ocular diseases, it is recommended that vancomycin be prescribed only if the patient has common risk factors for infection or in the recurrence or persistence of disease despite antibiotic treatment. Appropriate use of antibiotics reduces the development of additional resistant strains of organisms and the potential for adverse side effects. In serious infections sometimes broad-spectrum coverage does not include protection against MRSA, so accurate diagnosis is important. Empirical antibiotic coverage was initiated in 98% of ocular infections, but covered for MRSA in only 50% of cases. Fortunately, ocular isolates of MRSA were found to have 93.9% sensitivity to trimethoprim in a nationwide study conducted by the Ocular Tracking Resistance in US Today (TRUST).

Conclusion

MRSA should be suspected in atypical cases of orbital cellulitis and in cases of bacterial conjunctivitis that do not respond to standard topical therapy. In such cases, cultures should be obtained and therapy for MRSA considered. It remains uncertain if MRSA will produce significant ocular morbidity in epidemics of bacterial conjunctivitis in children, but it must be considered in all cases of atypical ocular and periocular infectious disease.

Acknowledgments

I would like to thank Lekha Ravindraraj, MD for her assistance in researching and contributing to this chapter.

Suggested Readings

Amato M, Pershing S, Walvick M, Tanaka SI. Trends in ophthalmic manifestations of methicillin-resistant *Staphylococcus aureus* (MRSA) in a northern california pediatric population. *J AAPOS*. 2013;17:243-247.

Freidlin J, Acharya N, Leitman TM. Spectrum of eye disease caused by methicillin-resistant *Staphylococcus aureus*. *Am J Ophthalmol*. 2007;144:313-315.

Haas J, Larson E, Ross B, et al. Epidemiology and diagnosis of hospital-acquired conjunctivitis among neonatal intensive care unit patients. *Pediatr Infect Dis J*. 2005;24:586-589.

Mathias MT, Horsley MB, Mawn LA, et al. Atypical presentations of orbital cellulitis caused by methicillin-resistant *Staphylococcus aureus*. *Ophthalmol*. 2012;119:1238-1243.

Rutar T. Vertically acquired community methicillin-resistant *Staphylococcus aureus* dacryocystitis in an infant. *J AAPOS*. 2009;13:79-81.

Vazan DF, Kodsi SR. Community-acquired methicillin-resistant *Staphylococcus aureus* orbital cellulitis in non-immunocompromised child. *J AAPOS*. 2008;12:205-206.

Walvick MD, Amato M. Ophthalmic methicillin-resistant *Staphylococcus aureus* infections: sensitivity and resistance profiles of 234 isolates. *J Community Health*. 2011;36:1024-1026.

HOW DO I MANAGE BLEPHARITIS AND CHALAZIA?

Rudolph S. Wagner, MD and Nicole Pritz, MD

Various lumps and bumps may appear on the eyelids of children. *Blepharitis* is a chronic inflammation of the eyelid margins and is a common cause of external ocular irritation. Patients may complain of burning, itching, light sensitivity, and foreign body sensation. Children may show signs of general ocular discomfort and rub their eyes frequently. These symptoms and eyelid crusting are usually worse in the morning. Frequently, a dermatological condition, such as seborrheic dermatitis, atopic dermatitis, or acne rosacea, is the underlying cause of chronic blepharitis. Therefore, it is vital for physicians to carefully examine the skin of patients with eyelid inflammation to rule out an associated systemic disorder.

Blepharitis can be classified according to anatomic location: *anterior blepharitis* affects the base of the eyelashes and the eyelash follicles, and *posterior blepharitis* affects the meibomian glands and gland orifices. Anterior blepharitis can be further divided into *staphylococcal* and *seborrheic* forms. In staphylococcal anterior blepharitis, colonization of the eyelids by bacteria, most commonly *Staphylococcus aureus*, leads to scaling and crusting around the base of the eyelashes (Figure 23-1). The seborrheic variant is characterized by mild erythema and thickening of the eyelid edges and formation of greasy flakes along the lid margins.

Posterior blepharitis, also called *meibomitis*, is caused by meibomian gland dysfunction. Meibomian glands are modified sebaceous glands located within the tarsal plates of the eyelids that are responsible for secretion of the oily layer of the tear film (Figure 23-2). Posterior blepharitis is characterized by hyperemia of the eyelid margin and telangiectatic blood vessels. White, foamy discharge may be seen along the lower eyelid margin. Meibomian orifices can become inspissated or plugged with thickened, waxy secretions.

Developing a regular routine of eyelid hygiene is essential in the treatment of blepharitis. This is often difficult in preverbal children, and their caregivers will play a major role in their

Wagner R. *Curbside Consultation in Pediatric
Ophthalmology: 49 Clinical Questions* (pp 109-112)
© 2014 SLACK Incorporated

Figure 23-1. Child with chronic staph blepharitis and ulcer on the inferior temporal cornea near the limbus.

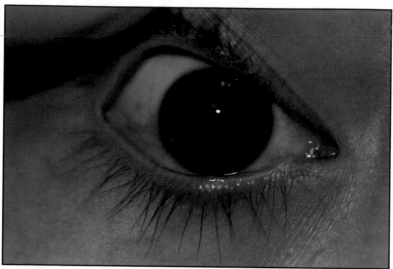

Figure 23-2. Drawing of the upper eyelid showing the various glands.

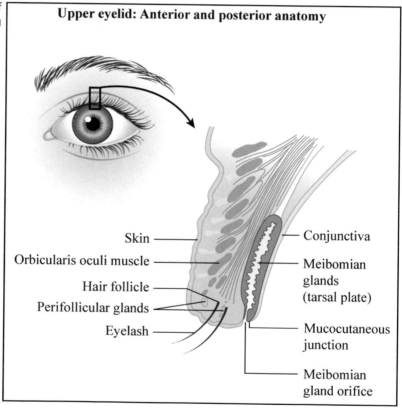

Upper eyelid: Anterior and posterior anatomy

Skin

Orbicularis oculi muscle

Hair follicle

Perifollicular glands

Eyelash

Conjunctiva

Meibomian glands (tarsal plate)

Mucocutaneous junction

Meibomian gland orifice

therapy. They should be instructed to apply a clean washcloth warmed with water to the eyelids for approximately 10 minutes at least twice daily to soften adherent encrustations and warm the meibomian secretions. It is important to remind caregivers to avoid using compresses that are so hot that they burn the skin. Lid hygiene can be accomplished by lightly massaging the eyelids to express meibomian secretions. Patients or caregivers can clean the eyelid by gently rubbing the base of the eyelashes using either diluted baby shampoo or commercially available eyelid cleaner.

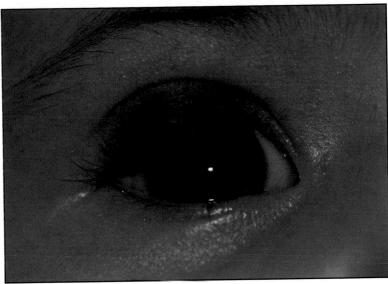

Figure 23-3. A chalazion on the right upper eyelid with external skin changes.

A topical antibiotic, such as bacitracin ophthalmic or erythromycin ointment, can also be used to reduce the bacterial load. Topical corticosteroids may be helpful in patients with marked inflammation but should be prescribed with caution because steroids may exacerbate conditions such as herpetic keratitis and can elevate the intraocular pressure, leading to glaucoma. Recently, there has been an increased interest in the role of polyunsaturated fatty acids in the management of blepharitis. Studies have provided evidence that dietary supplementation with omega-3 fatty acids in patients with meibomian gland dysfunction is effective in improving both symptoms and objective findings, such as a decrease in lid margin telangiectasias and meibomian gland blockage. This therapy may prove useful in children with chronically evolving chalazia.

In children, the front part of the eye can become sensitive to the bacteria that grow on the eyelid margins. This can lead to ocular surface inflammation, conjunctivitis, keratitis, corneal ulcers, and scarring. These children will present with chronic red eyes and may have visible white lesions on the corneal surface, particularly at the limbus. Therefore, early detection and appropriate treatment can prevent permanent damage and possible vision loss. It is important for a child to see an ophthalmologist if he or she develops a reduction in vision, intense sensitivity to light, or increasingly watery eyes.

One of the most common eyelid lesions presenting in children is a *chalazion*. This is a noninfectious, chronic, focal inflammation of the eyelid. The most common cause is blockage of a meibomian gland, which produces the lipid component of the tear film. The oily material exits from small duct openings along the eyelid margin. If the meibomian gland or duct becomes obstructed, the oily secretion backs up into the gland and stimulates a granulomatous inflammatory reaction in the surrounding tissue.

On examination, the patient may have a firm, mobile, painless nodule on the eyelid (Figure 23-3). Typically, the eye is white and quiet. Multiple chalazia may be seen involving one or more eyelids or eye lashes. Several predisposing factors, including patients with eye strain due to uncorrected refractive errors, repetitive rubbing of the eyes, and chronic blepharitis, are associated with recurrent chalazia.

Small chalazia may resolve spontaneously. Conservative treatment involves warm compresses and lid hygiene in an attempt to reopen the meibomian gland pore and allow the lipid material to drain, decompressing the chalazion. In some children, the compresses will result in the chalazion draining externally through the skin. If, despite continued treatment, the chalazion does

Figure 23-4. Acute hordeolum with cellulitis on the right lower eyelid.

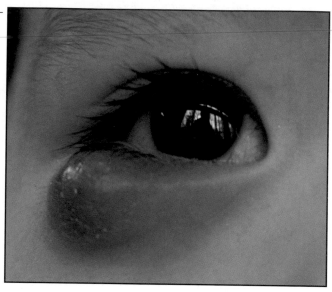

not reduce in size, the patient should be referred to an ophthalmologist for consideration of incision and curettage. In most cases, this will require surgery under general anesthesia, so parents should be instructed to diligently adhere to the prescribed therapy in an attempt to avoid surgery. Occasionally, an intralesional injection of steroid is performed instead of minor surgery, but this is difficult to perform in young children.

Another common eyelid mass in children is a *hordeolum*, which is the result of an acute bacterial infection of an eyelid gland. An *external hordeolum*, also known as a *stye*, is an acute, localized, pyogenic infection of the glands of Zeiss, which are small sebaceous glands associated with eyelashes. An *internal hordeolum*, which is less common, is a focal abscess of a meibomian gland. Patients usually present with a red, inflamed, edematous, and tender eyelid (Figure 23-4).

Hordeola are typically self-limited and will either spontaneously rupture and drain or be absorbed within several weeks. Both internal and external hordeola can be treated with warm compresses approximately 4 times per day. Concurrent treatment with topical antibiotic ointment is appropriate. Systemic antibiotics should be reserved for the development of preseptal cellulitis.

In all young children with any type of mass in the eyelid, it is crucial to monitor for partial occlusion of the visual axis or distortion of the globe causing astigmatism. Therefore, it is important to check the visual acuity of children with large eyelid lesions. If a decrease in vision is found, referral to an ophthalmologist is necessary to prevent the development of amblyopia.

Suggested Readings

American Academy of Ophthalmology. *Basic and Clinical Science Course. External Disease and Cornea: Section 8, 2009-2010*. San Francisco, CA: American Academy of Ophthalmology; 2009.

Macsai MS. The role of omega-3 dietary supplementation in blepharitis and meibomian gland dysfunction (an AOS thesis). *Trans Am Ophthalmol Soc.* 2008;106:336-356.

McCulley JP, Dougherty JM, Deneau DG. Classification of chronic blepharitis. *Ophthalmology.* 1982;89:1173-1180.

Stevens A, Lowe J. *Human Histology. 3rd ed.* Philadelphia, PA: Elsevier/Mosby; 2005.

SECTION V

STRABISMUS

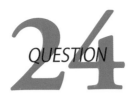

HOW CAN I DIFFERENTIATE A TRUE STRABISMUS FROM A PSEUDOSTRABISMUS?

Scott E. Olitsky, MD and Paula Grigorian, MD

Pseudostrabismus is common in infants and young children because the bridge of the nose is wide and flat, and the extra skin (epicanthal folds) that will generally disappear with time covers the white of the eyes, making the eyes appear crossed. These epicanthal folds are common in Down syndrome as well as in Asians and Native Americans. There are other less common causes of pseudostrabismus, such as that seen in children with a history of severe retinopathy of prematurity with ectopic maculae.

Although a complete eye examination would be able to differentiate true strabismus from pseudostrabismus, a few simple tests can be performed by the primary physician as well.

We will describe our approach to a patient who is referred with concerns of eye misalignment (Figure 24-1).

Parents of patients with pseudostrabismus often hand me a cell phone picture where the child looks slightly off center, making one eye appear crossed. It is important to review the pictures for the symmetry of the light reflex. In a reliable picture, the child should be looking straight at the camera, otherwise the red reflexes or the pupillary light reflexes seem asymmetric, giving the false appearance of strabismus or even leukocoria.

The simplest test is to shine a penlight in the child's eyes (Figure 24-2). The light reflected off the smooth convex surface of the cornea creates the corneal light reflex in the middle of the pupil (actually immediately behind the iris plane). This is the Hirschberg test. If the eyes are straight, the corneal light reflexes should be symmetrical, directly in the center of the pupil, or slightly nasal. This works even in the squirmiest, most uncooperative kids.

The Bruckner test is another way to assess eye alignment. By looking through the direct ophthalmoscope at both eyes simultaneously, you get information about the light reflexes, the red reflexes, refractive errors, media opacities, and pupil size (Figure 24-3). Photoscreeners are new,

Wagner R. *Curbside Consultation in Pediatric Ophthalmology: 49 Clinical Questions* (pp 115-118)
© 2014 SLACK Incorporated

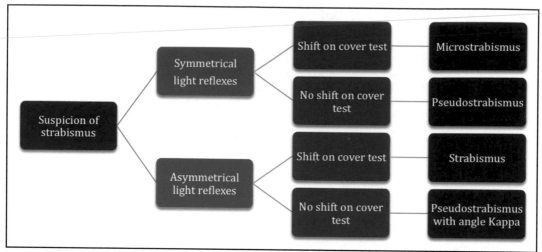

Figure 24-1. Examination diagram: clinical steps in examining patients with suspicion of strabismus.

Figure 24-2. Young patient with epicanthal folds and large nasal bridge appears to have crossing. Notice the symmetrical corneal light reflexes in the center of the pupil, demonstrating perfect alignment of the eyes.

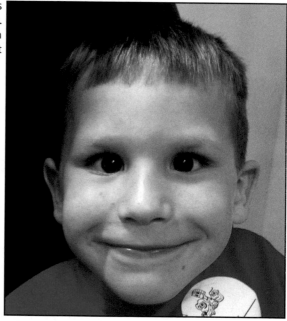

expensive devices that work on the same principle. They are cameras that take pictures of the red reflex of the eyes and analyze them for symmetry.

The previously mentioned tests are easy but not perfect. The tests may miss small degrees of strabismus that can be visually significant. They may also fail to detect cases of intermittent strabismus. In addition, if the visual axis does not go through the center of the pupil, the corneal light reflex would be displaced nasally or temporally, giving a false positive test (Figures 24-4 and 24-5). This disparity between the line of sight and the anatomic axis of the eye (the line that goes through the center of the pupil) is called *angle Kappa*. Patients with angle Kappa have pseudostrabismus and are not in need of treatment. The angle Kappa may be a family feature, or it may be caused by an ectopic, dragged macula like that seen in patients who have had severe retinopathy of prematurity.

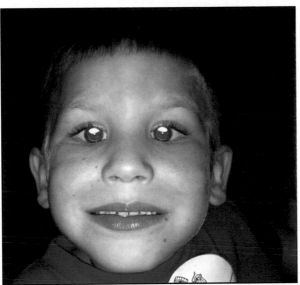

Figure 24-3. Pupillary red reflexes appear symmetrical, demonstrating good alignment of the visual axes.

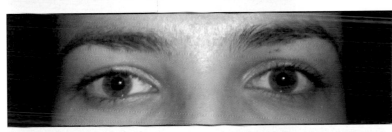

Figure 24-4. Patient with positive angle Kappa. Notice the asymmetrical light reflexes with the right reflex displaced nasally.

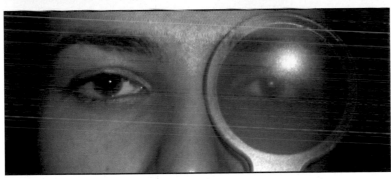

Figure 24-5. Same patient as in Figure 24-4. At cover test, the eyes do not demonstrate any refixation movements because the visual axes are already aligned.

To best demonstrate normal alignment, the gold standard is the cover test. The examiner covers one eye at a time and looks for any shift of the uncovered eye. The cover test is best performed with the child fixating on an object to make certain that any movement of the uncovered eye is due to strabismus and not due to lack of concentration (Figures 24-6 and 24-7). A toy or a movie can be used to capture the child's attention. The visual axes are well aligned if you do not see any refixation movements during the test.

Because pseudostrabismus can coexist with intermittent strabismus, it is important to do a full eye examination, including a cycloplegic refraction that may reveal high refractive errors as a cause of accommodative esotropia.

At the conclusion of these tests, it should be possible to tell the parents if a real strabismus is present. When we see a patient with pseudostrabismus, we reassure the parents that the child

Figure 24-6. Young patient with crossing of her left eye.

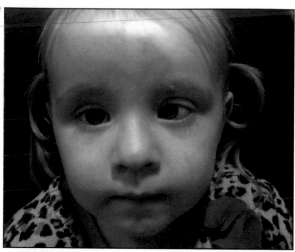

Figure 24-7. Cover test used to demonstrate the presence of strabismus. When the right eye is covered, the left eye takes fixation, changing position from crossed to straight.

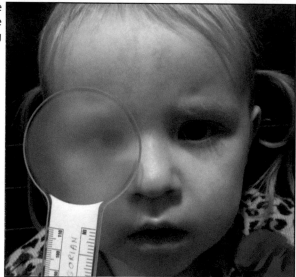

will outgrow the condition as his or her face grows and the nose develops, lifting up the extra skin that covers the corners of the eyes. If there is room for doubt, a follow-up examination may be warranted. In addition, it is important to tell the parents that true strabismus can develop in a child with pseudostrabismus. If there are changes that concern the parents at a later time, the child should be seen again.

Suggested Readings

American Association for Pediatric Ophthalmology and Strabismus. Pseudostrabismus. http://www.aapos.org/terms/conditions/88. February 2, 2014.

Arnoldi K. Case corner: pseudostrabismus: when are you sure? *Am Orthopt J.* 2005;55:162-165.

Jacobs HB. Pseudostrabismus: an audit. *Br J Ophthalmol.* 1978;62(11):763-764.

Pritchard C, Ellis GS Jr. Manifest strabismus following pseudostrabismus diagnosis. *Am Orthopt J.* 2007;57:111-117.

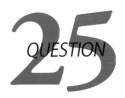

WHAT IS THE DIFFERENTIAL DIAGNOSIS OF A CHILD WHO COMPLAINS OF DOUBLE VISION, AND HOW DO I MANAGE IT?

Scott E. Olitsky, MD and Nicholas R. Binder, MD

Diplopia in the pediatric population can be a diagnostic challenge, and it is important to understand because several life-threatening conditions can present as diplopia. Part of the challenge lies in the fact that not all pediatric patients will complain of diplopia in the classic sense, especially younger patients. Younger patients may display nonspecific changes in behavior such as perceived clumsiness, inability to perform previously mastered motor skills, or frustration/agitation with visual-motor tasks. Patients younger than 18 months generally will not experience diplopia in the presence of ocular misalignment because of rapid neurological adaptation and resulting suppression of the deviated eye. Older children with chronic ocular misalignment also will not experience diplopia for the same reason. Therefore, a child complaining of diplopia will likely be preschool age or older and have an acute onset of symptoms. Another possible presentation would be parents bringing their child because they have noticed a new eye deviation, or abnormal head position or see that their child is closing one eye.

The 3 most important initial questions are as follows:

1. What was the acuity of onset?

2. Is the diplopia monocular or binocular?

3. Is the diplopia horizontal or vertical?

Acute Versus Chronic

Acuity of onset is important because acute diplopia often warrants an expedited work-up and immediate referral to the appropriate specialists. As mentioned above, a child with a chronic ocular misalignment usually does not experience diplopia; therefore, the simple fact that a child is complaining of diplopia usually implies an acute onset. Causes of acute binocular diplopia are listed in Table 25-1 and include cranial nerve palsies, orbital mass lesions, orbital inflammations/infections,

Wagner R. *Curbside Consultation in Pediatric
Ophthalmology: 49 Clinical Questions* (pp 119-122)
© 2014 SLACK Incorporated

Table 25-1

Differential Diagnosis of Acute Binocular Diplopia

Cranial Nerve Palsies (III, IV, and/or VI)	Orbital Disease	Muscular and Neuromuscular Disease
Intracranial infection (encephalitis, meningitis)	Rhabdomyosarcoma	Inferior rectus entrapment following floor fracture
Intracranial mass	Capillary hemangioma	Complications following eye muscle surgery
Increased intracranial pressure	Dermoid cyst	Orbital myositis
Head trauma (CN IV>VI>III)	Lymphoma	Botulism
Post-viral (usually CN VI)	Metastatic disease	Guillain-Barré syndrome (Miller Fisher variant)
Severe otitis media with mastoiditis (CN VI)	Infection and inflammation	Myasthenia gravis (rare in children)
Posterior communicating artery aneurysm (CN III)	Orbital cellulitis +/- subperiosteal abcess	Muscular dystrophies
Uncal herniation (CN III)	Thyroid eye disease (Graves' disease)	Some metabolic diseases
Multiple sclerosis	Orbital pseudotumor	
Hypertensive emergency		
Cavernous sinus thrombosis		
Migraine headache (rare)		

Abbreviation: CN, cranial nerve.

and diseases affecting the extraocular muscles. Chronic ocular misalignments in children more commonly represent a primary strabismus and call for a nonurgent referral to an ophthalmologist. Also, ocular misalignments manifesting within the first 6 months of age (in the absence of other findings) usually represent a primary strabismus and can be referred to ophthalmology within a few weeks (sooner than older children because the consequences of ocular misalignment on visual development progress more rapidly in the infant population).

Monocular Versus Binocular

Monocular versus binocular diplopia is important to elucidate because the etiologies of the 2 groups are different. *Monocular diplopia* represents non life-threatening (but potentially sight-threatening) conditions, whereas *binocular diplopia* should raise a red flag. The child and/or parents usually will not volunteer this information, but it is easily determined in the office. Have the child cover one eye and ask if he or she still has double vision. Repeat the test for the other eye. If the diplopia continues with one eye covered, it is monocular. If the diplopia resolves with either eye covered, it is binocular. It is important to test both eyes because monocular diplopia will

Table 25-2
Differential Diagnosis of Monocular Diplopia

- Corneal abrasion
- Other corneal surface irregularity
- Polycoria (multiple openings in iris)
- Lens dislocation
- Severe dry eye
- High astigmatism
- Lens opacity (cataract)
- Some retinal pathology

resolve with one eye covered if the covered eye is the one with pathology. If the child complains of seeing more than 2 images, this indicates a monocular etiology as well.

Alternatively, Hirschberg's test can be used as an objective way to determine ocular alignment in a child brought in because of an eye deviation noted by the parents or one of the behavior changes described above. With the child fixating on a light source, the position of the corneal light reflexes is noted. When the light reflexes are centered over both pupils, alignment is normal. If the light reflex is centered over one pupil but not the other, a misalignment is present. Caution should be used in declaring the eyes to be straight by this method because small deviations are easily missed even by an experienced observer.

Monocular diplopia implies a primary ocular etiology such as corneal abrasion, other corneal surface irregularities, polycoria (multiple openings in the iris other than the pupil), lens opacities, lens dislocation, or certain retinal pathologies (Table 25-2). Binocular diplopia implies a disorder of ocular alignment caused by cranial nerve palsy, orbital mass, orbital inflammations/infections, and diseases affecting the extraocular muscles and necessitates more urgent work-up.

Horizontal Versus Vertical

If the diplopia is binocular in nature, it helps to further classify the symptoms as horizontal or vertical. In monocular diplopia, this further classification is somewhat irrelevant. Simply ask the patient if the 2 images are seen mostly side by side or mostly one on top of the other. Sometimes there will be a pause and a response like, "One is over here and one is over there," while pointing to objects in a diagonal orientation. If this is the case, try to prompt the patient to decide whether the more prominent component of his or her diagonal diplopia is—horizontal or vertical.

Horizontal diplopia can be caused by a cranial nerve VI palsy, which is accompanied by limitation of abduction of the affected eye. This is in contrast to an acute primary horizontal strabismus, which will have full range of motility. Cranial nerve III palsy will produce a primarily horizontal diplopia (although concurrent with a smaller vertical component) and is accompanied by limitation of adduction, elevation, and depression of the affected eye. Cranial nerve III palsy is also variably accompanied by ptosis and pupil dilation. A pupil-involving third nerve palsy is an emergency requiring urgent neuroimaging and should be considered secondary to an intracranial aneurysm until proven otherwise. Remember that if ptosis obscures the visual axis in a cranial nerve III palsy, no symptoms of diplopia will be present. Internuclear or supranuclear lesions such as those seen in demyelinating disease can also cause horizontal diplopia.

Vertical diplopia can be caused by a cranial nerve IV palsy and is much more subtle than cranial nerve III and VI palsies. Most patients with an acute cranial nerve IV palsy will present with a head tilt to the side opposite the palsy to eliminate their diplopia. Limitation of vertical eye movement is not prominent. Trauma resulting in an orbital floor fracture can occasionally lead to entrapment of the inferior rectus muscle and a restriction of elevation. This restriction is usually considerable and may be accompanied by vagal symptoms such as nausea/vomiting and bradycardia, as opposed to the smaller limitations of eye movement produced by large, swollen eyelids that accompany blunt trauma. Demyelinating disease such as multiple sclerosis can also lead to lesions causing vertical diplopia.

Many other conditions will variably produce horizontal, vertical, or oblique diplopia. Orbital mass lesions (and sometimes eyelid lesions) that are large enough to displace the eyeball will produce diplopia with an orientation dependent on the direction in which the globe is pushed. Careful observation of the position of one globe relative to the other (Is there proptosis? Does one eye sit higher or lower than the other?) is important, and if abnormalities are present, they require orbital imaging. Orbital cellulitis can inflame any of the extraocular muscles causing variable limitations in motility. Sometimes it will lead to a subperiosteal abscess which in turn can produce mass effect on the globe. Intracranial infections (meningitis, encephalitis, abscess) and mass lesions can cause various cranial nerve palsies. Demyelinating disease can cause any type of cranial nerve palsy. Cavernous sinus thrombosis, large pituitary tumors, and mass lesions at the orbital apex can cause multiple concurrent cranial nerve palsies. Other inflammatory processes, such as thyroid eye disease and orbital myositis, can inflame any of the extraocular muscles and lead to muscle fibrosis and restriction over the long term. Neuromuscular junction disorders, such as myasthenia gravis, botulism, and Guillain-Barré syndrome (Miller Fisher variant), can cause variable diplopia and often first present with ocular findings. Muscular dystrophies can occasionally lead to diplopia as well.

Conclusion

A systematic approach to the child complaining of double vision is crucial. The main decisions that need to be made are the timing of appropriate specialist referrals and whether imaging is required. In general, acute presentation and binocular nature of diplopia are red flags that require a high degree of suspicion for serious underlying pathology. Subacute presentation is less concerning. Monocular diplopia involves only primary ocular causes but still may necessitate prompt referral because some sight-threatening conditions are associated. The horizontal versus vertical nature of diplopia can help narrow the differential diagnosis.

Suggested Readings

Moore BD. Strabismus: detection, diagnosis, and classification. In: *Eye Care for Infants and Young Children*. Boston, MA: Butterworth-Heinemann; 1997.

Nelson LB, Olitsky SE. Strabismus disorders. In: *Harley's Pediatric Ophthalmology*. 5th ed. Philadelphia, PA: Lippincott Williams & Wilkins; 2005.

Wright KW. Common forms of strabismus. In: *Pediatric Ophthalmology for Primary Care*. 3rd ed. Elk Grove Village, IL: American Academy of Pediatrics; 2008.

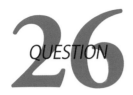

What Causes an Acute Esotropia, and How Should These Children Be Worked Up?

Leonard B. Nelson, MD, MBA

Acute acquired comitant esotropia (AACE) is an unusual presentation of an esodeviation that generally occurs in older children and adults.[1] It is characterized by the dramatic onset of a relatively large angle of esotropia with diplopia. Although there may be a brief period of intermittency, the esodeviation soon becomes constant. Double vision is an inconsistent finding because patients under the age of 9 years will develop suppression. If the acute esotropia is incomitant (meaning that it differs in lateral gaze positions), the child may develop a compensatory head position to avoid diplopia or may verbalize the presence of double vision. For example, a child with an acute right sixth cranial nerve or abducens nerve palsy may immediately develop a face turn to the right to keep the right eye in the adducted position to avoid double vision. In such cases, a diagnosis of increased intracranial pressure must be ruled out before a more benign condition like a post-viral sixth nerve palsy is considered.

Some cases of acute esotropia may actually be newly presenting accommodative esotropia. The finding of significant hyperopia by the pediatric ophthalmologist following cycloplegic retinoscopy supports this diagnosis. Children with accommodative esotropia usually have no other ophthalmologic findings and respond well to correction of hypermetropia with glasses.

Burian and Miller[2] have defined several types of AACE. Type I (Swan type) occurs after a period of occlusion of one eye, usually for amblyopia treatment. Type I AACE has also occurred after brief occlusion from the eyelid swelling secondary to blunt trauma. The refractive error is usually mildly hyperopic and does not affect the angle of deviation. The resulting esotropia is thought to be the result of an interruption of a previously well-functioning fusion system, causing a possible latent deviation to become manifest. In some cases, the deviation may spontaneously resolve, but in most cases the deviation remains constant, requiring treatment.

Wagner R. *Curbside Consultation in Pediatric
Ophthalmology: 49 Clinical Questions* (pp 123-125)
© 2014 SLACK Incorporated

In type II AACE (Franceschetti type), there is an acute onset of a relatively large angle of a comitant esotropia and diplopia. There is no obvious exogenous cause precipitating the esotropia. Again, the refractive error is usually mildly hyperopic. Therefore, like type I, an optical correction will not help reduce the deviation. Physical or psychological stresses have been suggested as the etiologic factor causing this type of AACE.[2] Some patients with type II AACE have a preexisting phoria or microtropia with reduced binocular vision before the onset of the tropia.[3] Other patients have normal binocular vision before the onset of acute esotropia.[3] Undoubtedly, which group these patients fall into will affect their surgical outcome in terms of a final sensory status.

Type III AACE is characterized by the acute onset of comitant esotropia in patients with uncorrected myopia of -5.00 diopters or greater.[1] The esotropia is typically at distance fixation but orthophoric at near fixation. The occurance of type III AACE presumably is caused by physical or mental stress. Some of these patients may initially present with a small angle of esotropia, often 10 prism diopters or less, but over a period of time the esodeviation becomes constant and quite large.[3] In many cases, the amount of myopia is high, and the esotropia becomes constant with near fixation as well.[3]

AACE often presents as a dramatic and alarming condition. These patients should have complete ophthalmological and neurological examinations with a careful history to rule out such conditions as cyclic esotropia, divergence insufficiency, paretic strabismus, and myasthenia gravis, any of which may also present acutely.[1] Any patient who presents with the acute onset of esotropia should evoke the question of whether the strabismus is a possible sign of a serious intracranial abnormality.[3] It is important to determine if the deviation is comitant or incomitant. If an acute esotropia is incomitant, it must be considered a sixth nerve palsy until proven otherwise. Most neuropathic or myopathic causes of strabismus present as an incomitant deviation.[3] However, having an acute esotropia that is comitant does not rule out the possibility that an underlying serious intracranial abnormality may exist. There are numerous reports of patients with acute-onset esotropia that are comitant who have an associated serious intracranial abnormality.[3] Tumors of the brainstem, cerebellum, pituitary region, and corpus collosum have all been reported with AACE.[3] Therefore, no single type of brain tumor or area of the brain can account for all the cases of AACE associated with intracranial abnormalities.[3]

The exact understanding of the etiology of AACE associated with some patients who, after extensive neurological evaluation, are found to have an intracranial abnormality is unknown. How is an ophthalmologist to approach a patient with AACE? If there are any potential neurological symptoms or findings, such as headaches, papilledema, or sudden change in functionality, immediate neurological investigation is necessary. Any associated nystagmus found in a patient with AACE should prompt an immediate neurological evaluation.[3] AACE with neurological abnormalities often presents with bilateral superior oblique muscle overaction and an A pattern.[4] Therefore, the absence of these findings might help the ophthalmologist distinguish between patients with AACE who do and do not have associated neurological abnormality.

If the ophthalmic examination is otherwise negative and a neurologic physical examination is normal, it is unclear whether further work-up, including computed tomography or magnetic resonance imaging, should be performed. Invasive studies, tensilon, and neuroradiologic testing in young children are not without risks. This is an important question that currently remains unanswered until further prospective studies are performed.

Patients with AACE who are found to have no neurological abnormalities should be treated initially with a hyperopic correction if it is at least +1.50 diopters in each eye. If after a period of time the esotropia is not reduced to within 8 prism diopters with the hyperopic correction, then strabismus surgery should be performed.[4] The potential for a reestablishment of binocular vision and high-grade stereopsis is excellent in many of those patients. Of course, the binocular status of these patients prior to their AACE is an important factor in their final binocular outcome.

However, binocular vision can be restored even in some patients in whom the interval of the onset of the esotropia and surgical procedure is delayed.[4] Most of these patients will have had normal binocular vision prior to the onset of AACE.

References

1. Clark AC, Nelson LB, Simon JW, et al. Acute acquired comitant esotropia. *BJ Ophthalmol.* 1989;73:636-638.
2. Burian HM, Miller JE. Concomitant convergent strabismus with acute onset. *Am J Ophthalmol.* 1958;45:55-64.
3. Hoyt CS, Good WV. Acute onset concomitant esotropia: when is it a sign of serious neurological disease? *Br J Ophthalmol.* 1995;79:498-501.
4. Sturm V, Menke MN, Knecht PB, et al. Long-term follow-up of children with acute acquired concomitant esotropia. *JAAPOS.* 2011;15:317-320.

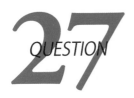

WHY DO SOME CHILDREN WITH ESOTROPIA NEED SURGERY WHILE OTHERS ONLY NEED GLASSES?

Patrick A. DeRespinis, MD, FACS, FAAP, FAAO

Esotropia, or the inward misalignment of one or both eyes, is a form of strabismus commonly seen in children. Although there are many forms of esotropia, the 2 most common types are accommodative esotropia and nonaccommodative esotropia (Figure 27-1). Congenital or infantile esotropia is a form of nonaccommodative esotropia present in children under the age of 1 year. In this section, I will frequently cite congenital esotropia when referring to nonaccommodative forms of esotropia, although nonaccommodative esotropia can also be acquired at a subsequent time. Accommodative esotropia requires the use of eyeglasses, and nonaccommodative esotropia requires surgery.

When a 6-month-old child is sent to my office with the diagnosis of inturned eyes, my approach is to first ascertain that the problem is a real one. A good percentage of infants sent to a pediatric ophthalmologist's office with the diagnosis of esotropia actually have pseudostrabismus. This condition mimics a true turn because infants have immature facial features, and the flat nasal bridges and prominent epicanthal skin folds cover the medial aspect of the conjunctiva, making the eyes appear closer together. I also carefully examine the eyes to rule out pathology, particularly those problems that could affect the vision and potentially cause a turn (eg, sensory esotropia). When more serious causes of strabismus (eg, retinoblastoma or cataracts) have been eliminated, it is important to distinguish accommodative esotropia from nonaccommodative forms of strabismus (eg, congenital esotropia) because each type has a different treatment modality.

Congenital esotropia usually becomes evident before 1 year of age. The amount of turn is usually significant (eg, greater than 30 prism diopters). Congenital esotropia can be classified as a syndrome because it has many associated components, including nystagmus, amblyopia, disassociated vertical deviations, V- and sometimes A-patterns, and poor fusion, often with absent stereopsis.[1] The child is typically neurologically intact. The deviation is usually equal at both near

Wagner R. *Curbside Consultation in Pediatric Ophthalmology: 49 Clinical Questions* (pp 127-130) © 2014 SLACK Incorporated

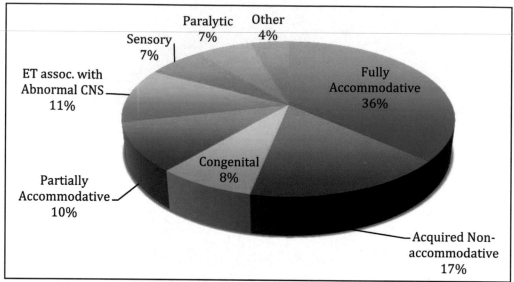

Figure 27-1. Incidence of esotropias in childhood. (Adapted from Greenberg A, Mohney B, Diehl N, Burke J. Incidence and types of childhood esotropia. *Ophthalmol.* 2007;114[1]:170-174.) Abbreviations: ET, esotropia; CNS, central nervous system.

and far. In congenital esotropia, although the turn does not vary much with accommodation, a dilated retinoscopic examination is necessary to ascertain the child's refractive error. Most infants with congenital esotropia do not require the use of eyeglasses unless there is a significant underlying refractive error.

The majority of infants younger than 1 year of age are hyperopic (farsighted) because their eyes are not fully developed and the axial lengths are shorter than those of an adult.[2] Pediatric ophthalmologists are unlikely to give small amounts of farsighted correction to treat the large amounts of strabismus usually seen in congenital esotropia. Getting an infant to wear eyeglasses is not an easy prospect, and small amounts of refractive correction are not likely to affect a change in a child with congenital esotropia. If the young child has moderate levels of farsightedness, the ophthalmologist will occasionally prescribe eyeglasses to eliminate any accommodative component in the turn (partially accommodative esotropia). If surgical correction is contemplated, this refractive error may affect the amount of surgery performed on the patient. Even after surgery to correct an infantile esotropia, a farsighted child may require the use of eyeglasses for an undetermined period of time.

Accommodative esotropia is a form of strabismus that involves the vergence centers in the brain stem and the focusing system in the human eye. It usually presents in children between the ages of 2 and 4 years. It does so for a number of reasons. The child's lens system can handle large amounts of farsightedness at an early age (approximately 14 diopters), but as the child grows older, this ability slowly diminishes. A child loses some of this ability even by the age of 2, and this combined with increased visual demands and deficient divergent fusional abilities can uncover the underlying accommodative esotropia.

There is an intimate relationship between accommodation and convergence, both having the goal to focus and align, respectively, the images on the eye's visual center (fovea). When a normal child focuses on an image, the lens changes shape determined by the distance to the object (accommodation).[3] At the same time, the eyes converge, and this convergence increases the closer the object comes to the face. When a child is farsighted, this convergence mechanism can overreact, and the child's eyes will turn inward at near and/or at far (Figure 27-2). By relieving the need to focus with the appropriate correction, we can often eliminate the turn. In some children,

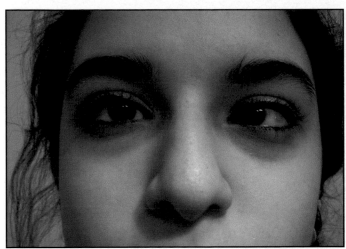

Figure 27-2. Child with uncorrected accommodative esotropia with high AC/A ratio.

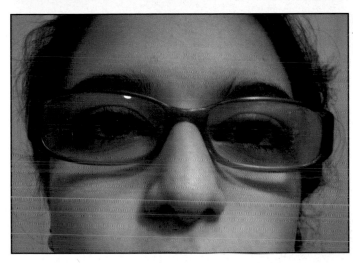

Figure 27-3. Accommodative esotropia corrected with eyeglasses and bifocal lenses.

even after the total amount of refractive correction is prescribed, a turn can still be present at near fixation (high accommodative convergence/accommodation [AC/A] ratio). These children may also require the use of bifocal lenses to eliminate the turn at near (Figure 27-3). As previously mentioned, children with a partially accommodative esotropia may even require surgery if the total amount of turn is not adequately reduced by eyeglasses. All of these treatments may also be performed in conjunction with occlusion therapy if it is determined that one eye does not see as well as the other (amblyopia). It is also important to remember that many farsighted children may not have strabismus. These children may or may not require eyeglasses depending on the amount of farsightedness.[4]

Although we are trained as surgeons, pediatric ophthalmologists would much rather treat a child medically if that is what the situation dictates. If we can treat the condition with eyeglasses and get the necessary outcome, this is preferred over putting a child under anesthesia. But what are the ophthalmologist's goals? There are many variables to consider. First and foremost, we want to preserve the child's vision. If esotropia is present, there is a strong chance amblyopia will develop, particularly if one eye is favored. We also want to optimize fusion and promote the development of normal depth perception (stereopsis) if possible. This can only occur when the eyes are properly aligned and the images on the retina are equally focused. A child with strabismus can also face psychosocial and developmental problems if the condition is not adequately treated.

I find there is a great deal of confusion among parents who want to know why their child has to wear glasses while another child had surgery and no longer has a turn. If accommodative esotropia patients have surgery that should not have been performed, consecutive exotropias may develop, which may lead to multiple unnecessary surgeries. Also, some children with accommodative esotropia eventually outgrow their turns over time as their visual systems mature. We have to understand that there is a different approach to a turn that requires surgery (congenital esotropia) and a turn that requires eyeglasses (accommodative esotropia). In the end, the only important consideration is that patients receive timely and thorough treatment to assure they achieve an optimal visual outcome.

References

1. Costenbader FD. Infantile esotropia. *Trans Am Ophthalmol Soc*. 1961;59:397.
2. Cook RC, Glasscock RE. Refractive and ocular findings in the newborn. *Am J Ophthalmol*. 1951;34:1407.
3. Donders FC. *On the Anomalies of Accommodation and Refraction of the Eye*. Translated by W.D. Moore. London, England: The New Sydenham Society; 1984.
4. DeRespinis PA. Eyeglasses: why and when do children need them? *Pediatr Ann*. 2001;30(8):457-459.

IS THERE AN OPTIMAL AGE FOR STRABISMUS SURGERY?

Scott E. Olitsky, MD and Luke Rebenitsch, MD

Strabismus is a common eye problem encountered in children, affecting between 2% and 5% of the preschool population.[1] Simply put, it is a misalignment in any field of gaze, and its presentation varies greatly. It can be constant or intermittent, and it can be manifest at distance and/or near fixation. The word is derived from the Greek word *strabismo*, meaning "a squinting," which dates back to the famous Greek geographer, Strabo.

When determining how and when to manage patients with strabismus, it is important to distinguish the type that affects your patient. To simplify, we will divide strabismus into the following 4 categories: congenital, intermittent, acquired, and paralytic. For the sake of ease and scope, we will not discuss less common forms of strabismus. It should also be noted that strabismus surgery in children has a long list of potential complications, and conservative management should be used when appropriate (Table 28-1). However, it should also be remembered that surgery, while considered a treatment of last resort by many parents, may indeed be the only appropriate treatment in many cases.

Of equal, if not greater, concern in managing patients with strabismus is amblyopia. This condition, in which the visual cortex never "learns" to use an eye, is a complication of strabismus that is paramount in the management of strabismus. This complication may even develop after surgical correction. It has been shown that amblyopia can be effectively treated both before and after realignment through penalization of the "good" eye throughout the first decade. However, aggressive patching, parental compliance, and evaluation are all much easier to perform prior to surgery. Therefore, we recommend treatment of amblyopia prior to surgical realignment.

Wagner R. *Curbside Consultation in Pediatric Ophthalmology: 49 Clinical Questions* (pp 131-136)
© 2014 SLACK Incorporated

Table 28-1

Complications of Strabismus Surgery

Less Serious	Serious
Unsatisfactory postoperative alignment	Slipped extraocular muscle
Conjunctival inclusion cyst	Anterior segment ischemia
Suture granuloma	Orbital cellulitis
Preseptal cellulitis	Endophthalmitis
Perforation of sclera*	Perforation of sclera*

*The perforation of the sclera is not always a serious complication and many times only leaves an insignificant chorioretinal scar.

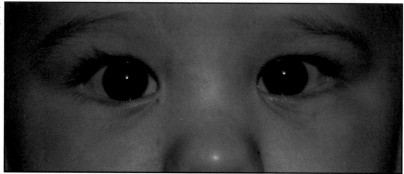

Figure 28-1. Pseudo-esotropia. This child has a flat nasal bridge and prominent epicanthal folds. Note the corneal reflex is central in both eyes.

Congenital Strabismus

Congenital strabismus is a common disorder. When evaluating a new patient for strabismus, you must differentiate from pseudostrabismus, an apparent crossing. This "disorder" affects as many as 50% of infants brought to the ophthalmologist by parents concerned about crossed eyes. The appearance is caused by a flat and broad nasal bridge, prominent epicanthal folds, and/or a narrow interpupillary distance (Figure 28-1). It is important to note that although there is no true deviation at this time, strabismus can still develop. The child should be evaluated if the condition does not improve.

By definition, the age of onset for congenital strabismus is between birth and 12 months. There have been opposing views in the past as to when is best to treat these patients. Until the 1960s, surgery was rarely performed before age 2 years because most surgeons felt that it was impossible to obtain functional improvement in these patients. This was proven to be incorrect.

Currently, most strabismus surgeons advocate surgery prior to 1 year of age. This gives the best chance to develop binocular vision. However, surgery in older children, and even adults, can still provide this functional improvement. There are few, if any, who obtain perfect binocular vision; however, the earlier the surgery is performed, the more likely the patient is to develop at least rudimentary binocular vision. This becomes important because those with a degree of stable binocular vision have been shown to be 50% less likely to develop strabismus again over a 20-year period.[2]

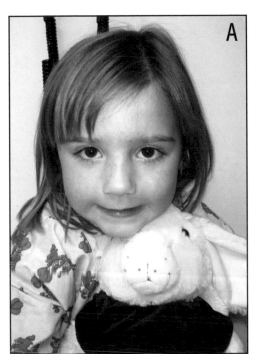
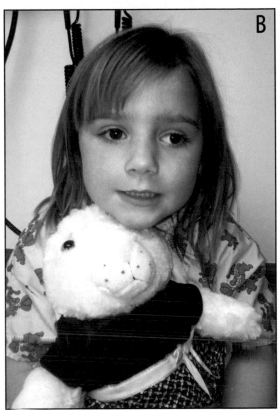

Figure 28-2. Intermittent exotropia. (A) The corneal reflex is in the center of both corneas, indicating straight eyes. (B) The reflex is not central in the right eye, indicating exotropia.

Intermittent Strabismus

In intermittent strabismus, there is a tendency for a manifest deviation, or "drifting" of the eyes, yet the strabismus is not always present. The most common form of intermittent strabismus is intermittent exotropia, which is the most common form of childhood strabismus (Figure 28-2). This deviation usually occurs between 6 months and 4 years of age. The deviation is usually greater at distance than near and generally has a natural progression in its severity. In the beginning, there is an intermittent loss of fusion ("drifting") at distance. The natural history of this disorder is a progression to total loss of fusion at distance followed by loss of fusion at near.

Throughout the early stages, there is no suppression of vision, and diplopia can often be elicited. Luckily, amblyopia rarely develops in these patients during the early stages. As the patient progresses, there is a development of suppression of an eye, and surgery is indicated. Timing of surgery is controversial. Studies have shown the cure rate is higher when the patient is younger than 7 years of age and has had the disorder for fewer than 5 years.[3] It may be most important to base the need for surgical intervention on the frequency of the strabismus. Most surgeons will suggest surgery when the deviation occurs a large portion of the day.

Acquired Strabismus

There are multiple etiologies to an acquired strabismus, the most common of which is an accommodative esotropia. When the crossing distance is fully corrected with eyeglasses, the patient can be observed and many times eventually weaned from glasses. If the deviation is fully corrected, surgery may be necessary.

Other etiologies for acquired strabismus include trauma, mass, idiopathic, and palsy. The most important aspect in the evaluation is the determination of cause. Once the etiology for the acquired strabismus has been determined and the deviation is constant and unlikely to improve, surgery is generally indicated to prevent amblyopia, improve a compensatory head position, and/or restore binocular vision.

Paralytic and Syndromic Strabismus

Paralysis of extraocular movement includes those of the third, fourth, and sixth cranial nerves. According to a study at the Mayo Clinic, the order of incidence for cranial nerve palsy for the pediatric population is the following: fourth, sixth, and third.[4] Strabismus due to palsy is further differentiated into acute or congenital etiologies and treated accordingly. When acute, an underlying mechanism should always be elicited, because it could be resultant of trauma, neoplasm, vascular, syndromic, or idiopathic.

The treatment of palsy varies by age of onset and etiology. A congenital palsy will rarely improve (aside from an occasional sixth). Initial management includes alternating patching and observation of head position, an indication of normal visual development. Earlier surgery is indicated when there is a lack of normal visual development (ie, amblyopia) or severe ptosis as in a thirrd nerve. In a fourth nerve palsy, in addition to improving head position, there is evidence that earlier surgery prevents facial asymmetry, and surgery is indicated earlier (Figure 28-3). In an acute setting, we generally wait 6 months before performing surgery to allow for spontaneous resolution or stabilization.

When the etiology of strabismus is syndromic, as in Duane's or Brown's, the management is directed toward alignment in straight-ahead gaze and improved head position. As with palsies, evaluation of normal visual development is important when determining the timing of surgery.

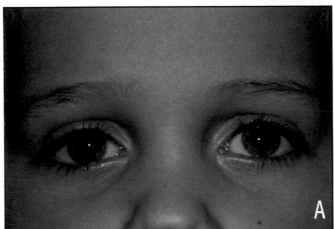

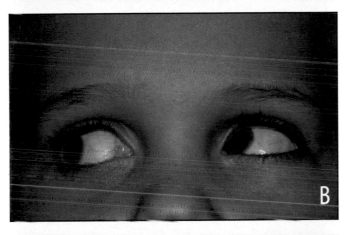

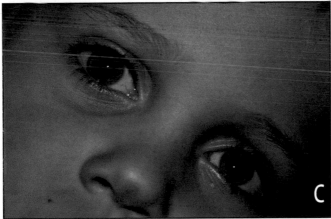

Figure 28-3. Left superior oblique palsy. (A) There is a left hypertropia, (B) increasing as the patient looks to the right (C) and when tilting the head to the left.

References

1. Graham PA. Epidemiology of strabismus. *Br J Ophthalmol.* 1974;58:224-231.
2. Arthur BW, Smith JT, Scott WE. Long term stability of alignment in the monofixation syndrome. *J Pediatr Ophthalmol Strabismus.* 1989;26:224-231.
3. Abroms AD, Mohney BG, Rush DP, et al. Timely surgery in intermittent and constant exotropia for superior sensory outcome. *Am J Ophthalmol.* 2001;131:111-116.
4. Richards BW, Jones FR, Younge BR. Causes and prognosis in 4,278 cases of paralysis of the oculomotor, trochlear and abducens cranial nerves. *Am J Ophthalmol.* 1992;113:489-496.

Suggested Readings

Harley R, Nelson L, Olitsky S. *Harley's Pediatric Ophthalmology.* 5th ed. Philadelphia, PA: Lippincott Williams & Wilkins; 2005:143-200.

Lorenz B, Brodsky M. *Pediatric Ophthalmology, Neuro-ophthalmology, Genetics.* Berlin, Germany: Springer-Verlag; 2010.

Tychsen L. Can ophthalmologists repair the brain in infantile esotropia? Early surgery, stereopsis, monofixation syndrome, and the legacy of marshall parks. *J AAPOS.* 2005;9(6):2005: 510-521.

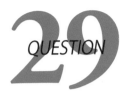

WHAT ARE THE CAUSES OF OCULAR TORTICOLLIS?

Scott E. Olitsky, MD and Florin Grigorian, MD

Ocular torticollis refers to an abnormal head position that is ocular or visual in nature. It is important to differentiate it from nonocular torticollis because ocular torticollis can usually be treated effectively, and failure to identify ocular causes and treat them in a timely manner can be deleterious to the visual or musculoskeletal systems. For these reasons, torticollis that does not have an obvious nonocular nature should be assumed ocular until proven otherwise. Referral to a specialist versed in identification and management of ocular causes of torticollis is advisable early in the process of the evaluation of torticollis.

What Are the Causes of Ocular Torticollis?

In general, ocular torticollis serves as a compensatory mechanism, and in this situation it is called *compensatory head position*. It can serve to increase visual acuity, obtain binocular vision, or center the visual field relative to body position. Alternatively, it may arise from primitive muscular tonus reaction to unequal visual input. Miscellaneous other compensatory and noncompensatory mechanisms are implicated in rare conditions.

Differential Diagnosis of Ocular Torticollis

Differential diagnosis is simplified by the high association of head tilt with contralateral superior oblique palsy. The 3 classic causes of ocular torticollis—nystagmus, strabismus, and refractive errors—together with eyelid ptosis encompass the vast majority of the differential diagnosis.

Wagner R. *Curbside Consultation in Pediatric Ophthalmology: 49 Clinical Questions* (pp 137-142) © 2014 SLACK Incorporated

Finding the etiology could still be a daunting task because there are a multitude of other cases. Moreover, finding the etiology is rendered more complicated by the presence of conditions with multifactorial ocular and nonocular causes for torticollis (eg, Down syndrome). There is also the possibility of longstanding abnormal head position to persist as habitual musculoskeletal deformity despite appropriate treatment and resolution of ocular torticollis.

To develop a differential diagnosis, it is useful to divide the abnormal head position into 3 types: head tilt, face turn, and chin elevation or depression. Particular types of strabismus, nystagmus, or refractive errors are associated with 1 of the 3 types of abnormal head positions, although they could be implicated in all 3 types. Still other causes are associated with only one type of head position (eg, ptosis is associated with chin up position). Table 29-1 summarizes the differential diagnosis of ocular torticollis.

HEAD TILT

The main ocular cause for a *head tilt* is a contralateral superior oblique palsy. This compensatory head position is used to eliminate double vision by placing the eyes into a position where the weak superior oblique muscle has to do the least amount of work (Figure 29-1). Nystagmus can also cause a head tilt in children with infantile nystagmus and a torsional null position. Caution should be exercised when attributing a head tilt to infantile nystagmus; confirmation can be obtained by demonstrating an increase in intensity of the nystagmus when tilting the head in the opposite direction. *Spasmus nutans* is a special form of nystagmus that is associated with a head tilt and head oscillation. *Ocular tilt reaction* is a neurologic or othologic condition that occurs when unilateral injury of the vestibular system creates a subjective tilt. Ocular tilt reaction can produce ocular head tilt, ocular torsion, and misalignment, which are not compensatory mechanisms to maintain binocular vision. Torticollis, epiphora, and photophobia can be presenting signs of a posterior fossa tumor that can be attributed to a combination of ocular tilt reaction with compression of the trigeminal nerve. Finally, uncorrected or poorly corrected refractive error could be implicated in an ocular head tilt. This etiology of abnormal head position could be diagnosed and treated early during ophthalmological examination by performing a refraction but it may be hard to identify otherwise. This is another reason why it is appropriate to have an ophthalmologist involved in the evaluation of a child with torticollis.

FACE TURN

The main differential diagnoses of a face turn are incomitant strabismus and nystagmus with a null point in lateral gaze. In both cases, there is a worsening of the condition with opposite head turn. Refractive errors that are not fully corrected in straight ahead gaze can result in a compensatory face turn to help increase vision. Other causes that are associated with a face turn include congenital homonymous hemianopsia, cortical visual insufficiency, gaze deviation or gaze palsy, and congenital ocular motor apraxia.

VERTICAL HEAD POSITION

Abnormal vertical head position is further subdivided in chin up and chin down positions to help in formulating a differential diagnosis. For chin up positions, the principal diagnosis is lid ptosis, either unilateral or bilateral. For bilateral ptosis, the head inclines back to clear the visual axis, and in unilateral ptosis, the head position ensures binocular vision. In the latter situation, the cessation of abnormal head position signifies the occurrence of amblyopia and the need to initiate amblyopia treatment. A restrictive vertical strabismus may also cause chin up or down positions.

Table 29-1

Differential Diagnosis of Ocular Torticollis

Head Tilt	Face Turn	Vertical Head Position
Superior oblique palsy—frequent cause of head tilt, rarely can cause head turn	Noncomitant strabismus—restrictive (eg, orbital fracture, thyroid ophthalmropathy, tumor, postoperative scar, excessive resections)	Congenital ptosis—unilateral or bilateral
Congenital nystagmus—can cause other type of abnormal head position	Noncomitant strabismus—paralytic (eg, CN 6 palsy, CN 3 palsy, slipped muscle, Duane's syndrome)	Horizontal strabismus with A or V pattern
Spasmus nutans—particular type of nystagmus; head tilt part of the defining triad; head turn can rarely be seen	Infantile esotropia—head turn more frequent than other abnormal head positions	Congenital nystagmus with vertical null point or with A or V pattern
Dissociated vertical divergence	Congenital nystagmus—head turn more frequent than other abnormal head positions	Other types of nystagmus—convergence retraction (chin up), downbeat nystagmus (chin down)
Infantile esotropia—associated with other types of abnormal head position	Other types of nystagmus—periodic alternating	Noncomitant strabismus—restrictive (eg, orbital fracture with entrapment, congenital fibrosis of EOM, thyroid ophthalmopathy, orbital tumor)
Plagiocephaly—can cause superior oblique dysfunction, hence head tilt	Congenital homonymous hemianopia	Noncomitant strabismus—paralytic (eg, trauma, monocular elevation deficiency)
Refractive errors	Horizontal gaze palsy	Vertical gaze palsy
Lens subluxation	Tonic gaze deviation	Tonic gaze deviation
Ocular tilt reaction—vestibular dysfunction with tilted sense of vertical	Monocular vision loss	Altitudinal visual field defect
	Eccentric fixation—macular heteropia in ROP, macular scar, macular dystrophy	Overlooking
	Cortical visual insufficiency	Refractive errors
	Congenital ocular motor apraxia	
	Refractive errors	

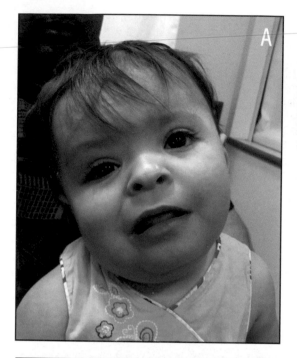

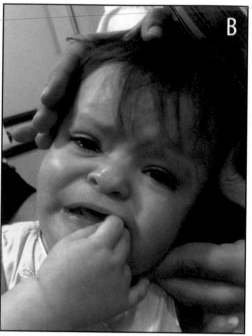

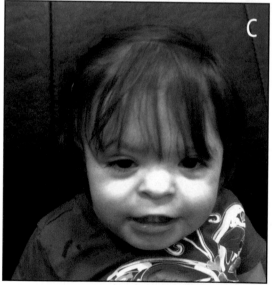

Figure 29-1. Child with left superior oblique palsy. (A) Compensatory head position with tilt to opposite side. (B) Forced tilt toward the side of palsy brings upward deviation of the left eye that in turn brings diplopia and strong resistance from child. (C) Improved head position after extraocular muscle (EOM) surgery.

Congenital fibrosis syndrome can present with a combination of ptosis and fixed down gaze, chin up position being compensatory for both (Figure 29-2). Nystagmus with a vertical null point is yet another cause of vertical head position, either chin up or down.

Management in the Clinic

A history should be obtained to attempt to establish the probable time of onset. Significant abnormal head position that starts right after birth is suggestive of nonocular, musculoskeletal

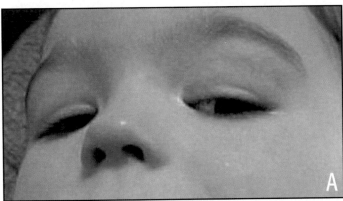

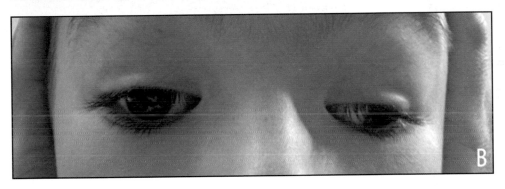

Figure 29-2. Child with congenital fibrosis of EOM with difficult elevation in both eyes, bilateral ptosis, and exotropia. (A) Marked compensatory head position with predominant chin up position and secondary head tilt and face turn. (B) Aspect of the eyelids and alignment in forced straight-ahead position.

origin of torticollis (ie, congenital muscular torticollis), whereas onset a few months after birth is suggestive of compensatory head position. Any old photographs or video recordings may help to date the onset and severity and should be reviewed so that unnecessary imaging may be avoided.

The approach to the child with torticollis that may be ocular in nature starts with a general inspection to characterize the position of the head: head tilt right or left, head turn right or left, and vertical head position with chin up or down. Although more than one abnormal head position can occur, if one dominant type of ocular torticollis is identified, this can help in the differential diagnoses. Head tilt, head turn, and abnormal vertical head position each have distinct sets of underlying diagnosis, although overlap exists. Prolonged observation of the patient is advisable to determine if some visual tasks elicit the compensatory head position.

Palpation of the neck can be helpful to differentiate between nonocular and ocular torticollis. A tight muscle in the neck or palpation of a mass along the muscle in the neck is highly suggestive of muscular torticollis. Assessing resistance to head repositioning can be used to separate ocular from nonocular torticollis and to differentiate among various types of ocular torticollis. Stiff resistance is suggestive of a musculoskeletal anomaly, although it can be encountered in cases of ocular torticollis when the child has a strong drive to maintain binocular vision. Lower resistance with a prompt return is suggestive of compensatory head position, likely ocular in nature. Minimal resistance with maintenance of the new head position is suggestive of habitual head position.

Monocular occlusion is a powerful tool to isolate ocular from nonocular torticollis. Improvement in head position with monocular occlusion suggests a compensatory ocular etiology aiming for improvement in binocularity. However, there are causes of ocular torticollis that do not improve with occlusion—nystagmus being the most common.

Visual acuity recording in the preferred head position should be followed by visual acuity in forced straight or opposite head position. Uncorrectable decreased vision should prompt a search for subtle nystagmus.

The ophthalmologist will use examinations of motility, visual fields, refraction, and the fundus as part of the evaluation for possible ocular torticollis. Eye movement recordings can confirm the presence of nystagmus that escaped confirmation during the clinical examination.

Finally, referring patients to experts in other specialties is warranted when nonocular torticollis is suspected, and imaging is needed when serious pathology of the brain or orbit is suspected.

Suggested Readings

Brodsky MC. *Pediatric Neuro-Ophthalmology*, 2nd ed. New York, NY: Springer Science+Business Media LLC; 2010:443-464.

Kraft SP. Abnormal head postures in children: causes and management. In: Hoyt CS, Taylor D. *Pediatric Ophthalmology and Strabismus*, 4th ed. Elsevier Ltd; 2013:822-835.

Rubin SE, Wagner RS. Ocular torticollis. *Surv Ophthalmol.* 1987;3(6):366-376.

Shah AS, Hunter DG. Practical problems: abnormal head postures. In: Hoyt CS, Taylor D. *Pediatric Ophthalmology and Strabismus*, 4th ed. Elsevier Ltd; 2013:1030-1032.

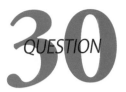

Do Eye Exercises Work in the Treatment of Strabismus?

Kyle Arnoldi, CO

There are few clinical situations in which eye exercises would be considered an ideal primary or exclusive course of treatment for strabismus. Exercises are more often used successfully as an adjunctive therapy in combination with optical, medical, or surgical management techniques. Eye exercises, also known as orthoptic exercises, can be beneficial under very specific circumstances but may be a futile, expensive, and generally harmless waste of time in some cases, and even contraindicated in others. Although "exercises" may sound benign, these techniques can be just as harmful as other treatment modalities if used inappropriately.

How Do Eye Exercises Work?

The mechanism that adjusts eye position, taking the globes from a position of rest to centered and aligned in the orbits, is the vergence system. Vergence is a type of bilateral disconjugate eye movement that is controlled by visuomotor centers and pathways in the cortex and brain stem. There are several complementary types of vergence that operate under different circumstances, in response to different stimuli, each with their own time course and with different roles to play in achieving and maintaining eye alignment.

Image disparity-driven vergence (also known as fast vergence) is triggered by the perception of identical images as slightly offset due to misalignment of the visual axes. The purpose of this type of vergence is to align the eyes and keep them straight to allow sensory fusion (the ability to coalesce images from each eye into a single perception). It is therefore sometimes referred to as motor fusion or fusional vergence. Motor fusion is also primed to compensate for the small misalignments that

Wagner R. *Curbside Consultation in Pediatric Ophthalmology: 49 Clinical Questions* (pp 143-146) © 2014 SLACK Incorporated

---

Table 30-1
Characteristics of the Ideal Candidate for Eye Exercises

- Age >5 years
- Horizontal eye misalignment
- Small to moderate misalignment
- Fair to good control (intermittent or latent deviation)
- History of normal binocular vision system and good visual acuity
- Normal extraocular muscles
- Normal ocular motor nerves
- Intact supranuclear pathways for eye movement

---

occur naturally as a consequence of normal eye movements and to respond to physiologic changes in eye position that occur gradually over the course of a lifetime.

When the fast vergence system is called upon habitually to make the same correction in eye position over an extended period of time, the brain responds by making an adjustment in the slow vergence system. Slow vergence is responsible for resetting the baseline eye alignment to reduce the pressure on the fast vergence system. A program of eye exercises takes advantage of the vergence system's malleability by simulating a small increase in the misalignment under controlled conditions to trigger a modification of the baseline eye alignment. In other words, "eye exercises" do not exercise the eyes or the eye muscles; they exercise the brain.

Stressing the fast vergence system with exercises over a long enough period of time can result in semipermanent changes in eye alignment. When the additional vergence demand is removed, however, the slow vergence system gradually adjusts to return the eyes to the original baseline position.

Under What Circumstances Would Exercises Be Helpful?

Motor fusion operates most efficiently when the eye misalignment is small and/or changing slowly; the individual is otherwise healthy, with good vision in both eyes and a history of normal binocular vision; and the individual has normal extraocular muscles, ocular motor nerves, and mature cortical vergence pathways. These are also the ideal conditions under which a patient would best respond to exercising the motor fusion system (Table 30-1). The patient who would most benefit from eye exercises as a primary method of management is the older child or adult with a small to moderate horizontal (preferably divergent) eye misalignment that is at least partially controlled by the patient's natural vergence ability. Unfortunately, only a small fraction of all patients with strabismus fit this description.

When the vergence system, extraocular muscles, or ocular motor nerves are abnormal due to injury, imbalance, or maldevelopment, or the motor fusion system is overloaded by a large angle and/or acute misalignment, a symptomatic strabismus that is unlikely to respond to exercising the disparity-driven vergence pathway may be the result. For example, a child younger than age 5 will not be able to understand the proper technique for most of the exercise regimens, and/or may not have the attention span required for daily practice. Moderate to large angle deviations or acute

Table 30-2
Limitations and Risks of Using Eye Exercises in the Treatment of Strabismus

- Significant delay to improvement or cure
- Reduced potential for full recovery of binocular vision if used in an unsuitable case
- Permanent double vision if used in an unsuitable case
- Temporary exacerbation of symptoms
- Increased risk of recurrence of deviation/symptoms
- Inability to cure strabismus

misalignments tend to overwhelm the vergence system. The vergence system is better equipped to compensate for horizontal misalignments, because these are much more common, although we have a limited range of vertical vergence. A strabismus that is uncontrolled or poorly controlled suggests that the vergence system is not sound, leaving no foundation on which to build better vergence ability with exercises.

This means that eye exercises are not appropriate as a primary treatment for most types of infantile or childhood-onset strabismus. Neither are they effective in most cases of ocular motor nerve palsy, brain injury (including cerebral palsy), congenital dysinnervation syndromes (such as Duane's syndrome), or abnormal orbital or muscle anatomy (such as in congenital craniofacial disorders) if used as the primary or exclusive treatment.

What Are the Disadvantages of Managing Strabismus With Exercises?

Table 30-2 lists the limitations and risks of using eye exercises in the management of strabismus. In the management of strabismus, time is of the utmost importance. Unfortunately, eye exercises do not have the immediate effect that optical, medical, and surgical treatments do because the vergence system needs a significant amount of time to adapt. Treatment with eye exercises alone will typically take weeks to months of daily work to register objective improvement. The delay to a cure is a significant problem because the longer the duration of strabismus, especially when it is constant, the less likely the patient can achieve a functional cure with any treatment strategy. This is particularly true for children because their robust neuroplasticity can so readily adapt to anomalous sensory input from misaligned eyes and prevent the development of a normal binocular vision system, even after the strabismus is repaired. Even in the adult patient with strabismus, minimizing the duration of misalignment increases the chances for full recovery of binocular vision. But whereas the child's strabismus should ideally be corrected within weeks of onset, the adult has more time before potential for recovery suffers.

Exercises are also contraindicated in some cases of childhood-onset constant strabismus because of the increased risk of intractable double vision. Early onset strabismus often leads to a maldevelopment of binocular vision, including coordinated binocular eye movements such as vergence. Exercising an abnormal system typically leads to undesirable functional outcomes.

Because of the nature of this type of treatment, when applied in a suitable case, the symptoms often become much worse before they begin to improve. Because eye exercises work by increasing the vergence demand even further on a system that is already being taxed, symptoms of eye strain, fatigue, or headache may be exacerbated.

The effect of treatment with exercise is temporary. To remain symptom free for a lifetime, the patient will have to periodically restart the training to maintain control.

Finally, eye exercises do not cure strabismus. The goal of this type of treatment is to help the patient attain better control over eye alignment, thereby relieving symptoms and reducing the risk of deterioration or recurrence of the deviation. For this reason, they are often most effective when prescribed in conjunction with optical or surgical techniques.

Conclusion

Eye exercises can be a useful adjunct in the treatment of strabismus if used judiciously in a suitable case with realistic treatment goals in mind. The ideal candidate is a healthy teen or adult patient with an intermittent or latent, small- to moderate-sized horizontal deviation and an otherwise normal visual system. The candidate must be persistent, patient, and able to tolerate some discomfort. The patient should also be diligent in monitoring his or her own symptoms to be ready and able to resume the exercises when necessary.

Suggested Readings

Abdi S, Rydberg A. Asthenopia in schoolchildren, orthoptic and ophthalmological findings and treatment. *Doc Ophthalmol.* 2005;111:65-72.

Eibschitz-Tsimhoni M, Archer SM, Furr BA, DelMonte MA. Current concepts in the management of concomitant exo-deviations. *Compr Ophthalmol Update.* 2007;8:213-223.

Helveston EM. Visual training: current status in ophthalmology. *Am J Ophthalmol.* 2005;140:903-910.

Luu CD, Abel L. The plasticity of vertical motor and sensory fusion in normal subjects. *Strabismus.* 2003;11:109-118.

Piano M, O'Connor AR. Conservative management of intermittent distance exotropia: a review. *Am Orthopt J.* 2011;61:103-116.

Thiagaraian P, Lakshminarayanan V, Bobier WR. Effect of vergence adaptation and positive fusional vergence training on oculomotor parameters. *Optom Vis Sci.* 2010; 87:487-493.

SECTION VI

GENERAL EYE COMPLAINTS

WHAT CAUSES LIGHT SENSITIVITY IN CHILDREN?

Javaneh Abbasian, MD and Brian J. Forbes, MD, PhD

Light sensitivity, also called *photophobia* or *photosensitivity*, is an unusual reaction upon exposure to light, usually the sun. Although most sun reactions typically involve the skin, the eyes can also be overly sensitive to light. Depending on its etiology, photophobia can manifest in numerous ways, including shutting the eyes, tearing, or avoidance of bright lighting conditions.

Causes

Many things can trigger light sensitivity. The easiest way to think about the causes is to break up the etiologies according to anatomic location.

CORNEA

The most common causes of photophobia are corneal in origin, with the most common problem in a photophobic child being a *corneal abrasion*, or a scratch on the surface epithelium of the cornea.[1] Often the child will have had a minor trauma with a toy or fingernail, after which the child will complain or show signs of pain and will have trouble opening the eye. Shining a light in the eye will also evoke tearing most of the time. Diagnosis is often made with the help of fluorescein dye and cobalt blue light (or Wood's lamp).

Although abrasions (Figure 31-1) are the most common corneal problem, any epithelial disruption can cause photophobia. *Keratitis*, or inflammation of the cornea, is caused by numerous pathogens and produces an irregular, irritating corneal surface. A feared cause of epithelial keratitis is herpes simplex virus, which can result in a typical dendritic keratopathy (Figure 31-2). This

Wagner R. *Curbside Consultation in Pediatric Ophthalmology: 49 Clinical Questions* (pp 149-153)
© 2014 SLACK Incorporated

Figure 31-1. Corneal abrasion seen as a fluorescent green defect of corneal epithelium. Fluorescein dye and Wood's lamp were used to visualize (cobalt blue light may be used as well).

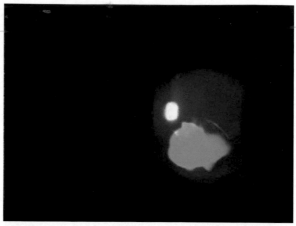

Figure 31-2. Herpes simplex branching dendrite seen with the aid of fluorescein dye and cobalt blue lamp.

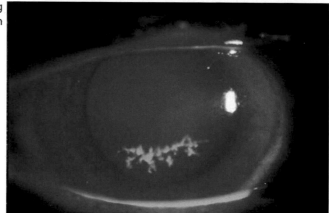

virus can also be diagnosed using fluorescein dye and should prompt an emergent referral to an ophthalmologist for evaluation and treatment.

Bacterial, fungal, and viral infections can also cause a keratitis, which can progress to corneal ulceration. This progression tends to occur in the setting of a trauma to the eye or in contact lens wearers. It can manifest with an extremely red eye with intense pain and a decrease in vision.

Chemical injury can also cause photophobia, and in the acute setting, an immediate saline flush should be initiated with the pH monitored after substantial irrigation has occurred. In addition, corneal foreign bodies, although uncommon in kids, should also be considered if plausible by history. Any history of trauma can lead to corneal scarring, which by itself can cause photophobia for years after the initial injury.

HEREDITARY DISEASE

One of the most important causes of true photophobia is *congenital glaucoma*.[2] As the intraocular pressure increases, the corneal diameter will enlarge, and this stretching causes breaks in Descemet's membrane (called *Haab's striae*). Resultant edema and corneal scarring can cause intense photophobia, a sign that is sometimes misinterpreted as nasolacrimal duct obstruction. Interstitial keratitis, an immune reaction seen in congenital syphilis, can also cause light sensitivity; other signs include hearing loss and peg-shaped teeth. Together with interstitial keratitis, these 3 signs are known as *Hutchinson's triad*.

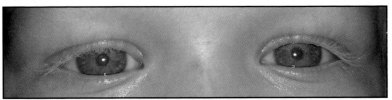

Figure 31-3. Transillumination defects seen in a child with albinism. Lack of iris stromal pigment allows the red reflex to shine through, giving the appearance of a pink-colored iris.

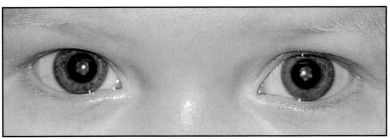

Figure 31-4. Posterior subcapsular cataracts seen centrally obscuring the pupil. This can be identified by observing the red reflex using a direct ophthalmoscope in a dimly lit room.

Aniridia and albinism (Figure 31-3) are also important causes of photophobia, both resulting from an inadequate barrier to light by the iris.[3] In aniridia, the lack of iris structure allows light to pass through the iris. Similarly, in albinism, although the iris is present, pigmentary loss prevents satisfactory filtration. Metabolic disease such as cystinoisis and tyrosinemia should also be considered where appropriate.

UVEA

Inflammation of the uveal tract can also cause photosensitivity. In simple iritis, anterior chamber cell and flare are important signs denoting inflammation. Childhood iritis can be infectious in origin, idiopathic, and/or traumatic. It is caused by many pathogens, including but not limited to Lyme disease, tuberculosis, or syphilis. An important inflammatory cause of uveitis is *juvenile idiopathic arthritis* (JIA), which can cause devastating sequelae and blindness if not properly recognized and treated, although the uveitis associated with JIA is only rarely associated with photophobia.

LENS

Partial lens opacities can cause light sensitivity, especially those opacities in the posterior aspect of the lens called *posterior subcapsular cataracts* (PSC) (Figure 31-4). These cataracts can be hereditary or associated with diabetes mellitus, radiation therapy, heavy steroid use, or various other less common etiologies. Photophobia has also been noted in patients with a partially subluxed lens (eg, patients with Marfan syndrome, homocystinuria, or Weill-Marchesani syndrome).

RETINA

Hereditary retinal dystrophies are usually seen in patients at birth and can present with severe photophobia, decreased visual acuity, and poor color vision.[4] Cone dystrophy leads to progressive dysfunction of cone cells in the retina, whereas congenital achromatopsia is nonprogressive but results in absent or severely abnormal cones. Whenever hereditary dystrophy is suspected, electro-physiologic testing should be conducted to confirm the diagnosis.

NEUROLOGIC

Meningitis and encephalitis are other important causes of light sensitivity. Both are seen in the context of other systemic abnormalities with the eyes presenting minimal concern. Optic neuritis, although uncommon in children, can cause light sensitivity and should be considered if other signs of optic nerve compromise are present (eg, decreased color, abnormal papillary reaction).

MISCELLANEOUS

Other causes of photophobia include medications, dilated pupils, sun allergy, and recent eye surgery. Strabismus itself can cause an apparent photophobia. For example, a child with intermittent exotropia may squint in sunlight to avoid diplopia, giving the appearance of photosensitivity.

How Is Light Sensitivity Diagnosed and Treated?

A physician can often determine the cause of the light sensitivity by the patient's medical history. Topics to cover include the following:

- Onset, duration, and previous history of photophobia?
- Age group of the child—infant, toddler, or adolescent?
- Intensity of light sensitivity—mild, moderate, or severe?
- History of recent trauma? Illicit history of foreign body if plausible.
- History of recent infection?
- History of contact lens use?
- Other medical problems, especially hereditary/metabolic?
- History of high-dose steroid use, radiation therapy, or prescription medications?
- Family history of eye disease?
- Eye pain? Tearing? Blepharospasm? Brow ache?

For example, a history of recent eye infection, the use of certain medications, or the presence of disease such as Marfan syndrome, can point to the underlying cause of light sensitivity. A careful eye examination is often needed to rule out uveitis or glaucoma (an intraocular pressure assessment is necessary if this is suspected). Examination with fluorescein dye and a Wood's lamp should also be done because corneal etiology is common. Direct ophthalmoscopy is also helpful to rule out disc edema or macular changes. Further examination and diagnostics by an ophthalmologist is always warranted in equivocal cases where a diagnosis is not obvious.

Treatment/Management

Treatment depends upon the underlying cause. In the case of a corneal abrasion, often antibiotic ointment will alleviate symptoms while the cornea heals. Patients with keratitis or corneal ulceration should undergo culture and sensitivity testing, as well as antibiotic therapy consistent with the pathogen suspected. If uveitis is suspected, a careful slit lamp and fundus examination will guide the differential diagnosis and subsequent ancillary testing. Patients are often treated with steroids and cycloplegic agents, but infectious etiologies should always be considered. In cases of lens dislocation or cataract, an evaluation by an ophthalmologist is necessary for refractive treatments or surgical management. In cases of hereditary or metabolic causes, collaboration with an ophthalmologist and/or geneticist is often valuable.

If neurologic causes are suspected, appropriate diagnostics could include neuroimaging or lumbar puncture with culture and sensitivities. A careful history and fundus examination with direct ophthalmoscopy will be important to guide these urgent diagnoses.

In cases of mild or moderate photophobia, dark glasses indoors or outdoors and avoidance of bright lighting conditions during the acute phase is often helpful. This may also be helpful in patients with albinism, aniridia, or hereditary retinal or metabolic disorders. If the light sensitivity is due to medication, switching to an alternative drug may be necessary.

Course of Light Sensitivity

Depending on the etiology of photophobia, the course of this symptom can vary. In patients with corneal abrasions, the photophobia will resolve with healing of the corneal epithelium. In contrast, in patients with corneal scarring from trauma or keratitis, these symptoms may become chronic. Similarly, in patients with hereditary or metabolic disease, photophobia may be a life-long problem. It is important to keep in mind that proper diagnosis is essential to educate patients about the course and management of light sensitivity. Where appropriate, referral to an ophthalmologist or a low-vision specialist can aid in diagnosis and treatment.

References

1. Rittichier KK, Roback MG, Bassett KE. Are signs and symptoms associated with persistent corneal abrasions in children? *Arch Pediatr Adolesc Med.* 2000;154(4):370-374.
2. Seidman DJ, Nelson LB, Calhoun JH, Spaeth GL, Harley RD. Signs and symptoms in the presentation of primary infantile glaucoma. *Pediatrics.* 1986;77(3):399-404.
3. Levin AV, Stroh E. Albinism for the busy clinician. *JAAPOS.* 2011;15(1):59-66.
4. Rajak SN, Currie AD, Dubois VJ, Morris M, Vickers S. Tinted contact lenses as an alternative management for photophobia in stationary cone dystrophies in children. *JAAPOS.* 2006;10(4):336-339.

QUESTION 32

DO REFRACTIVE ERRORS CAUSE HEADACHES?

Larry Frohman, MD

For many years, the question as to whether headaches can be caused by refractive errors (that require glasses) has been debated. The question is still not fully answered. One problem is that if you ask patients if they have headaches, the answer is commonly yes. In a study by Whittington [1] of more than 1400 consecutive patients presenting for refraction, 45% reported headache. In such studies, it is likely that the use of "headache" overlaps with the concept of asthenopia, which may be a nonspecific malaise of the eyes with use. To further analyze if headache may truly be caused by refractive error, we must first define what we mean by "headache."

Here, we are not referring to the primary headache syndromes defined in the 2004 International Classification of Headache Disorders-II (ICHD-2),[2] such as migraine, tension-type, cluster, and other related headaches. We are referring to what they describe as *headache related to refractive disorders*. In ICHD-2, headache related to strabismus is a different headache category. Fortunately, to further clarify whether headache may be related to refractive error, the ICHD-2 established the following formal criteria for establishing that a case of headache is indeed due to refractive error:

- That the headache is recurrent and mild and is in the frontal area and in the eyes themselves
- That there is an uncorrected or improperly corrected hyperopia, myopia, or astigmatism present
- That the headache and eye pain are temporally related to the refractive error, such as being absent on awakening and worsened by prolonged visual tasks without visual correction
- That the headache resolves, and does not recur, when given appropriate refractive correction

Thus, if we define the headache in this manner, the short answer is that there may be cases where mild headache may be related to a refractive error. However, for the majority of cases where refractive error is contemplated as the source of headache, especially when it does not meet the

Wagner R. *Curbside Consultation in Pediatric Ophthalmology: 49 Clinical Questions* (pp 155-157)
© 2014 SLACK Incorporated

ICHC-2 criteria, notably if the headache is severe, we cannot consider refractive error as the primary source of the headache. Several studies, including several that did not use the ICHD-2 to define the kind of headache to which they were referring, have tried to address this issue.

The problem with many of the studies is that they fail to account for the effect of superimposed strabismus on top of refractive error, and thus fail to show that it is uncorrected refractive error and not the misaligned eyes leading to the headache. Furthermore, they typically do not account for the placebo effect of receiving eyeglasses upon headache.[3]

In 2002, before the release of ICHD-2, Gil-Gouveia and Martins[4] asked the simple question: Is headache more frequent in those with or without refractive error? They found that the frequency of headache was equal in those who were found to have refractive errors and in those who were not, with some form of headache being present in about half of each group. They used an earlier headache classification with a similar definition of what they called "Headache Associated with Refractive Errors" (HARE). HARE was not seen in the control group but was seen in 6.6% of their study group, which was composed of people who self-presented to a refraction clinic (this use of a pool of patients who self-presented may lead to a bias and overestimation of the percentage of patients with refractive errors who have HARE, because those with HARE may be more likely to self-present than those who did not have HARE). Whereas headache frequency and headache severity did *not* correlate with the type of refractive error, the presence of HARE correlated with hyperopia but not with other forms of refractive error.[4]

What may be true is that refractive error may exacerbate the headache of those who already have headaches of nonrefractive origin. Among the patients in this study who had headache of any form, not just HARE, when those with refractive errors were given eyeglasses, 73% reported that their headaches were improved. To quote Gil-Gouveia and Martins[4], "In those with chronic headache, proper correction of refractive errors significantly improved headache complaints and did so primarily by decreasing the frequency of headache episodes." Interestingly, in the 7 patients who were found to have HARE, only 3 got headache improvement when given their glasses, perhaps indicating there was a second underlying cause of headache, reflecting the study's findings that half of patients with no refractive error reported headaches. The authors suggest HARE might be due to prolonged contraction of facial/periocular muscles in myopes squinting in an attempt to obtain a pinhole effect or, in presbyopes and hyperopes, from ciliary muscle strain from prolonged accommodation.

In a study performed in Turkey, 310 patients referred for headache were compared with 843 controls in terms of their refractive errors. A problem with this study is that this was not a random group of headache patients; they were already selected by having a negative assessment by neurology and otolaryngology, and all had already had some negative form of neuroimaging. The headaches met criteria 1 and 3 from the ICHD-2. The control group consisted of children referred for eye examinations for reasons other than headache, who did not have ocular disease known to cause headache, such as optic neuritis or acute glaucoma. Different and large numbers of children with strabismus, which, unfortunately, may have confounded the data from the study, were excluded from each group. Nonetheless, they found that children with headache had a 1.57 times risk of having a refractive error when compared with the control group. Yet, unlike the Gil-Gouveia and Martins[4] study, which found a possible association between headache and hyperopia, here it was astigmatism that was associated with increased incidence of headaches. Relative risk of headache did increase with severity of the refractive error. One of their highest associations was between a child having an improper refraction and the incidence of headaches.[5]

In a Dutch study, 487 children aged 11 to 13 years were examined and had headaches assessed via a survey tool. These children were unselected students from elementary schools. Seventy percent of these children reported headaches in the past year. The headaches were frequent in 37% of children and severe in 15%. In reviewing their data, which compared boys and girls, and right eyed versus left eyed refractive data (although in some data elements, there were barely statistically significant correlations), it is difficult to draw any conclusion about refractive error being a source of headache.[6]

The only way to potentially answer this question is to have 2 groups of study subjects: one that has significant uncorrected refractive errors and no other ocular problems, and one that does not have refractive errors. Divide each group into those who will be given their appropriate refraction and those who will be given either placebo eyeglasses or given eyeglasses with a predetermined error in the correction (eg, a 1-diopter undercorrection of myopia), and survey them for headaches before and after a period of eyeglasses use to ascertain if those with appropriate refraction had a significant decrease in the frequency or severity of headaches. This kind of study would be still be flawed but would be superior to those currently in the literature. Unfortunately, this study would be quite complex, and, due to the high incidence of headaches in the pediatric population, would require such a large pool of subjects that it would simply be impractical. Data mining of electronic medical records could perhaps shed some light upon the impact of proper eyeglasses correction upon headaches in the future.

For now, the following guidelines seem reasonable:

- Severe headaches, such as those that awaken a patient at night or are associated with nausea or vomiting, are not due to refractive errors.

- Syndromic headaches, such as migraines or cluster headache, should not be attributed to refractive error.

- Because receiving an improper refraction may be correlated with onset of headaches, the primary caregiver should be asked if the onset of the headaches seems to correlate with the receiving of a new correction.

- Prolonged squinting may cause a kind of muscle contraction headache, so it is reasonable to ask if the patient or family is aware of frequent squinting.

- Headaches that are related to visual effort are typically worse later in the day and, in school-children, may be worse on school days. If such a history is obtained and the headache is frontal or in the eyes and is mild, it is reasonable (in the absence of other physical examination or historical clues pointing to other causes) to consider whether the headache may be related to a refractive error.

References

1. Whittington TD. *The Art of Clinical Refraction*. London, England: Oxford University Press; 1958:11-18.
2. Headache Classification Subcommittee of the International Headache Society. The international classification of headache disorders. *Cephalgia*. 2004;24(1).
3. Gael E, Gordon G, Chronicle EP, Rolan P. Why do we still not know whether refractive error causes headaches? Towards a framework for evidence based practice. *Ophthal Physiol Opt*. 2001;21(1):45-50.
4. Gil-Gouveia R. Martins IP. Headaches associated with refractive errors: myth or reality? *Headache*. 2002;42(4):256-262.
5. Akinci A, Guven A, Degerliyurt A, Kibar E, Mutlu M, Citirik M. American Association for Pediatric Ophthalmology & Strabismus. *J AAPOS*. 2008;12(3):290-293.
6. Hendricks TJW, Brabander J, Van Der Horst FG, Hendrikse F, Knottnerus JA. Relationship between habitual refractive errors and headache complaints in schoolchildren. *Optom Vis Sci*. 2007;84(2):137-143.

Supported by a grant from Research to Prevent Blindness, Inc.

SECTION VII

TUMORS

How Do I Manage Periocular Hemangiomas? At What Point and to Whom Do I Refer?

Nina Ni, MD and Suqin Guo, MD

Infantile hemangioma (IH) is the most common periorbital and orbital vascular tumor of infancy, characterized by a hypercellular proliferation phase during the first year and followed by a long involutional phase over the subsequent 1 to 7 years. They can be bright red superficial capillary hemangiomas (historically referred to as strawberry hemangiomas) or present as purple masses that arise from deep within the reticular dermis and subcutaneous tissue (also known as *cavernous hemangiomas*). The first step is diagnosis, which is generally a combination of clinical judgment based on the above characteristics and imaging studies to rule out neoplasms. The differential includes other vascular and soft tissue growths such as tufted angioma, hemangiopericytoma, and fibrosarcoma. However, IH demonstrates a high flow pattern, asymmetry, and irregular acoustic features on Doppler ultrasonography, whereas solid tumors and vascular malformations exhibit low flow patterns. Further studies such as computed tomography, magnetic resonance imaging, or even biopsies are usually unnecessary. Referral to a specialist is generally only necessary if the diagnosis is in question or if the lesion is atypical.

Referral

Because hemangiomas will spontaneously regress over time, it would be appropriate to observe asymptomatic lesions through their natural course once the diagnosis has been established. However, periorbital lesions pose a unique concern because they occur during the pivotal phase of a child's visual system development. In addition to aesthetic considerations, a mass that occludes the visual axis and distorts the cornea can cause amblyopia and significant astigmatism, leading to lasting visual damage if not treated promptly. The incidence of amblyopia or permanent visual

Wagner R. *Curbside Consultation in Pediatric Ophthalmology: 49 Clinical Questions* (pp 161-164)
© 2014 SLACK Incorporated

loss resulting from complications such as astigmatism, strabismus, and mass effects can be as high as 60%.[1] Therefore, referral to ophthalmologists for early treatment is imperative in these high-risk periocular lesions. We suggest that every routine office visit include screening ophthalmologic examinations, and a referral to the ophthalmologist should be made for any of the following concerning signs associated with periocular hemangiomas:

- Failure to track
- Decreased visual acuity
- Inability to fully close the eyelids
- Misalignment of the eyes
- Lesions that occlude the visual axis or compress the globe
- Very rapid growth
- Ulceration/bleeding
- Diameter > 1 cm
- Deep tissue involvement

Management

There are several options in the ophthalmologist's armamentarium for the treatment of IH, and it is important for us to work together with pediatricians during the follow-up phase as well. A fairly new but effective treatment of hemangioma is the nonselective beta blocker propranolol, first reported by a group of French physicians in 2008.[2] Because the drug is systemic application and adverse effects can be severe even at the currently recommended low dose of 2 to 3 mg/kg/day, children should be monitored closely in conjunction with the treating ophthalmologist. There is no consensus guideline for baseline screening prior to starting propranolol treatment, but we advocate at least vitals, glucose, and electrocardiography (ECG). We work with pediatric cardiologists and obtain screening echocardiograms. We also recruit parents to perform home monitoring by educating them to recognize alarming signs and symptoms such as lethargy, poor feeding, wheezing, and bradycardia. There are several suggested treatment protocols, with some authors advocating initiation with gradual dose escalation up to 1 to 2 mg/kg/day divided in 2 or 3 doses, but we generally give the maintenance dose at onset.[3] Vitals will be monitored by the ophthalmologist 1 to 3 hours after each dose administration during the induction phase, in accordance with peak absorption time. Length of treatment is generally guided by clinical resolution of the hemangioma, although initial improvement has been noted within hours to weeks. During the course of treatment, patients may experience minor side effects such as sleep disturbances and gastrointestinal discomfort. Severe cardiovascular and pulmonary side effects are rare but have been reported; patients with symptomatic bradycardia, hypotension, or bronchospasm presenting to the pediatrician may rarely require cessation of treatment. Even subjective reports of vague symptoms such as agitation and fatigue could reflect underlying bradycardia or hypotension. Although hypoglycemia can occur, it is responsive to frequent feeding and we do not recommend routine finger stick glucose checks unless prolonged fasting is expected. At our institution, we have also been using the topical beta blocker timolol with good results for localized superficial periocular IH[3] (Figures 33-1 and 33-2). We have not yet encountered systemic side effects using topical timolol.

The most commonly encountered traditional treatments are steroids (intralesional injection or oral), surgery, and laser, all of which may cause side effects. The potential complications of intralesional steroids are largely confined to the realm of the ophthalmologist and include local skin toxicities such as hypopigmentation and fat atrophy, elevated intraocular pressure, and central

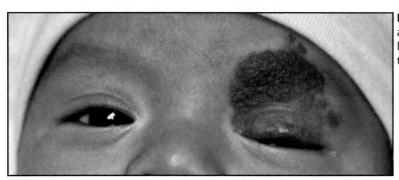

Figure 33-1. An infant with a large hemangioma on the left upper eyelid, occluding the pupil and visual axis.

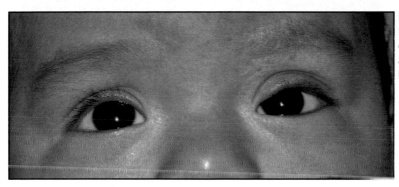

Figure 33-2. This baby's hemangioma is almost completely resolved after application of topical timolol solution for 4 months.

retinal artery occlusion. Although we have not seen adrenal dysfunction as a result of local treatment, rare cases have been reported and should be considered in symptomatic children presenting with a history of intralesional steroid injection.[4]

For large lesions that may require long-term oral steroids, there is a higher risk of systemic side effects that may result in more frequent pediatrician visits. In one study, even at doses of <3 mg/kg per day for 1 month, tapered over 2 to 3 months, most patients developed temporary cushingnoid faces, up to one-third of patients experienced height gain deceleration, and 29% experienced personality changes such as depressed mood, euphoria, insomnia, restlessness, and irritability.[5] A minority also experienced gastric irritation. However, parents can be reassured with the observation that the majority of these effects resolved with cessation of therapy. More serious risks include hypertension, adrenal cortical insufficiency, immunosuppression, and gastrointestinal bleeding, but these are more commonly seen in the high-dose steroids used with asthmatic or rheumatologic patients. If the side effects become intolerable or risks begin to outweigh the benefits, alternative treatments for the hemangioma should be discussed in conjunction with the ophthalmologist and the family.

In patients treated with surgery or laser, the standard postprocedural complications such as infection, bleeding, scarring, and hypopigmentation may be expected and the family should be forewarned. Immunomodulators such as cyclophosphamide and interferon-α are reserved as last-line treatments for vision- or life-threatening lesions because the treatments can last 1 year and side effects are quite significant. Besides reassuring parents about mild side effects such as fever and elevated liver function tests, the pediatrician must also carefully monitor for evidence of frequent infections and anemia due to myelosuppression, hepatotoxicity, and neurotoxicity (spastic diplegia).

Conclusion

Early referral to ophthalmology for the treatment of high-risk periocular hemangioma is essential to prevent permanent visual loss. Worrisome signs include decreased visual acuity, eyelid distortion, large or fast-growing lesions, and lesions that occlude the visual axis or compress the globe. Once a plan of treatment is initiated, with the most common being beta blockers, steroids, and surgery, we also work closely with the pediatrician to carefully monitor for possible side effects.

References

1. Lawley LP, Siegfried E, Todd JL. Propranolol treatment for hemangioma of infancy: risks and recommendations. *Pediatrc Dermatol.* 2009;26:610-614.
2. Léauté-Labrèze C, Dumas de la Roque E, Hubiche T, Boralevi F, Thambo JB, Taïeb A. Propranolol for severe hemangiomas of infancy. *N Engl J Med.* 2008;358(24):2649-2651.
3. Guo S, Ni N. Topical treatment for capillary hemangioma of the eyelid using topical beta-blocker solution. *Arch Ophthalmol.* 2010;128(2):255-256.
4. Weiss AH, Kelly JP. Reappraisal of astigmatism induced by periocular capillary hemangioma and treatment with intralesional corticosteroid injection. *Ophthalmol.* 2008;115:390-397.
5. Boon LM, MacDonald DM, Mulliken JB. Complications of systemic corticosteroid therapy for problematic hemangioma. *Plast Reconstr Surg.* 1999;104(6):1616-1623.

WHAT ARE THE MOST COMMON EYELID AND ORBITAL NEOPLASMS IN CHILDREN, AND HOW CAN I DIFFERENTIATE THEM?

Carol L Shields, MD

Neoplasms of the Eyelid

The eyelid can spawn both benign and malignant tumors. Most eyelid tumors in children are benign. The most common benign tumors include capillary hemangioma of infancy, eyelid nevus, kissing eyelid nevus, pilomatrixoma, neurilemoma, apocrine hydrocystoma, and, rarely, basal cell carcinoma. Each of these tumors has different clinical features, such as age of onset, color, effect on eyelid tissues, surface erosion, and prognosis.

Capillary hemangiomas of infancy are usually not present at birth but appear in the skin as a red vascular mass shortly thereafter and continue to grow for many months (Figures 34-1 and 34-2). *Kasabach-Merritt syndrome* is a condition where platelet sequestration by the hemangioma leads to hemolytic anemia, thrombocytopenia, coagulopathy, and early death. Posterior fossa, hemangioma, arterial lesions, cardiac abnormalities/aortic coarctation, and eye abnormalities (*PHACE syndrome)* occurs in children with large facial hemangiomas larger than 5 cm who may have brain hemangiomas, resulting in fatality. Treatment of capillary hemangioma of infancy is generally observation when it is not in the periocular region. However, when it is obstructing visual axis or causing strabismus, first line treatment includes propranolol 2 mg per kg given orally if the hemangioma is large or given topically if the hemangioma is flat. This tumor slowly involutes, sometimes leaving redundant skin changes.

Congenital eyelid nevi generally appear as a pigmented birthmark, occasionally with a hairy surface. When the upper and lower eyelids have similar lesions, it is termed a *kissing nevus*. The best time for management is when the child is 2 to 3 weeks old, with curettage of the superficial skin layers to remove the lesion. If this is not performed, this lesion extends deeper with time and is more difficult to remove, often requiring skin grafts at a later date.

Wagner R. *Curbside Consultation in Pediatric Ophthalmology: 49 Clinical Questions* (pp 165-169) © 2014 SLACK Incorporated

Figure 34-1. Cutaneous capillary hemangioma of infancy.

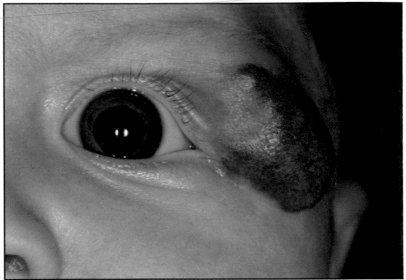

Figure 34-2. Cutaneous capillary hemangioma of infancy with extensive forehead and eyelid involvement as well as orbital involvement.

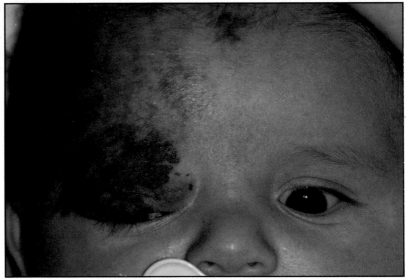

Pilomatrixoma is a tumor of the eyelid that occurs in children or young adults mostly under 10 years of age and involves the upper eyelid and brow most often. It appears as a solitary pink to purple nodular mass arising from a hair shaft and requires full excision (Figures 34-3 and 34-4). *Neurilemoma* appears as a yellow mass and can be nodular or plexiform. The nodular type can be resected, but the plexiform type can only be debulked.

Apocrine hydrocystoma is a tumor of the sweat gland (apocrine gland) and it has a bluish purple color. Surgical excision is warranted.

Lastly, basal cell carcinoma can occur in children. This is a rare occurrence and manifests usually as a nonhealing erosive lesion. You should search for the *Gorlin-Goltz syndrome*, an autosomal-dominant condition that predisposes patients to multiple basal cell carcinomas, particularly at a young age.

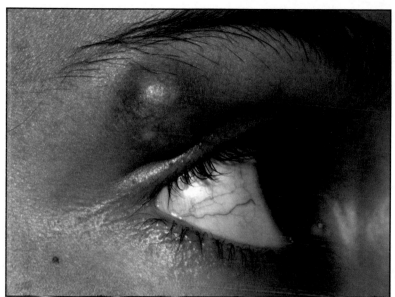

Figure 34-3. Eyelid pilomatrixoma.

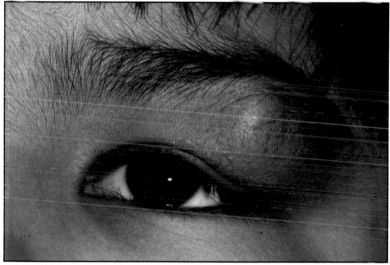

Figure 34-4. Eyelid pilomatrixoma.

Orbital Neoplasms

The most common orbital neoplasms in children include those of cystic, vascular, inflammatory, and myogenic origin. Cystic tumors mostly include the *dermoid cyst,* a benign congenital mass of misplaced epithelium within the orbit. A dermoid cyst is the fluid-filled structure and is lined most often by skin. If the cyst is located temporally in the orbit, it is lined by cutaneous skin and if medially located, it is lined by conjunctiva. Cysts appear as slow-growing, subcutaneous nodular masses, most often on the temporal orbital rim or eyelid. When palpated, they feel firm and not attached to the overlying skin. Dermoid or epidermoid cysts, depending on their pathologic diagnosis, are perhaps the most common benign orbital neoplasms seen in pediatrics. Surgical excision is warranted, because these lesions grow and occasionally rupture spontaneously.

Figure 34-5. Orbital lymph-angioma with hemorrhage.

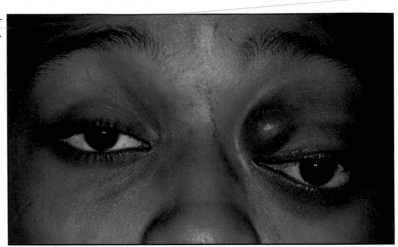

Figure 34-6. Orbitocon-junctival lymphangioma with hemorrhage.

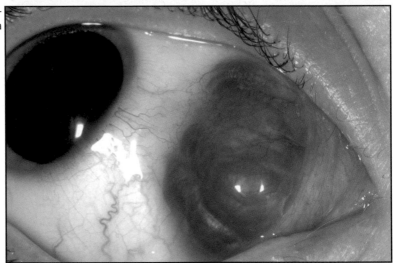

The most common vascular orbital tumors in children include capillary hemangioma and lymphangioma. Capillary hemangioma is seen in infants and gradually enlarges over time, producing progressive proptosis. These tumors often require surgical resection or systemic propranolol treatment. Lymphangioma generally does not enlarge over time but can hemorrhage, leading to massive abrupt proptosis (Figures 34-5 and 34-6). Drainage of hemorrhagic cysts of lymphangioma can be challenging. Complete resection of lymphangioma is often not possible.

The inflammatory pediatric orbital tumors include pseudotumor and its painful variant myositis. This is recognized by painful bouts of proptosis or disrupted ocular motility in a child or young adult. Treatment includes confirmation with CT or MRI, followed by institution of oral corticosteroids. If this plan is not successful, biopsy is necessary.

The last and perhaps most serious orbital tumor is *rhabdomyosarcoma*. These present as rapidly growing orbital masses with proptosis and often downward displacement of the globe (Figures 34-7 and 34-8). This malignancy represents approximately 5% of all orbital tumors in children and is the most common pediatric primary orbital malignancy. Although they can occur earlier, the average age of onset for rhabdomyosarcoma is 5 to 7 years. This malignancy carried a 70% mortality rate in the 1970s and currently carries only a 5% mortality rate as a result of

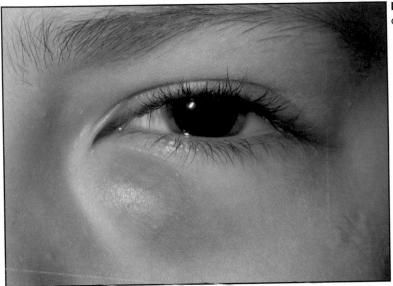

Figure 34-7. Orbital rhabdomyosarcoma.

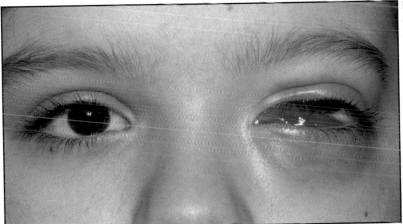

Figure 34-8. Massive orbital rhabdomyosarcoma.

improved therapy. Rhabdomyosarcoma is managed with precise imaging, followed by complete resection if possible. Once resected, the tumor undergoes staging and treatment, either with systemic chemotherapy or chemotherapy combined with radiotherapy.

Suggested Reading

Shields JA, Shields CL. *Eyelid, Conjunctival, and Orbital Tumors: An Atlas and Textbook*. 2nd ed. Philadelphia, PA: Lippincott Williams & Wilkins; 2008.

Support provided by the Eye Tumor Research Foundation, Philadelphia, PA.

WHAT CLINICAL FINDINGS SHOULD MAKE ME SUSPECT AN ORBITAL TUMOR, AND WHAT TYPES OCCUR IN CHILDREN?

Carol L. Shields, MD

Orbital tumors are relatively uncommon in children. Orbital tumors can produce features of proptosis, disrupted ocular motility, pain on eye movement, pain in the orbit, swollen eyelid, swollen conjunctiva, and generalized redness around the ocular region. Pupillary abnormalities such as a dilated pupil with an afferent papillary defect may occur if the optic nerve is compromised by the tumor. Children who present with symptoms of pain and redness most often manifest inflammation, such as preseptal cellulitis or orbital cellulitis. Rarely does pain and redness indicate an underlying malignancy. The most common malignancies to produce those symptoms include lacrimal gland malignancy and other malignancies that invade the perineural region. Other benign conditions can cause pain, including rapid proptosis from hemorrhagic lymphangioma. Most orbital tumors do not produce pain. They present quietly behind the child's eye with symptoms of proptosis, eyelid retraction, or swollen eyelid. In infants, the most common tumor is capillary hemangioma of infancy or orbital dermoid. They can be differentiated based on magnetic resonance imaging features showing the vascular enhancing mass of hemangioma versus the cystic mass with no internal enhancement of dermoid cysts. As patients age into their preteen years, the most common orbital tumors include pseudotumor, orbital myositis, lymphangioma (Figures 35-1 and 35-2), and rhabdomyosarcoma (Figures 35-3 and 35-4). These can be differentiated based on imaging features, with pseudotumor and myositis showing enhancement of the orbit diffusely or of the muscle, respectively. Lymphangioma shows multicystic mass with fluid-fluid levels on imaging. Rhabdomyosarcoma appears as a solid mass with diffuse enhancement. The management for these conditions differ in that the inflammatory conditions are managed with oral corticosteroids, the lymphangioma with resection or drainage of hemorrhage, and rhabdomyosarcoma with wide surgical resection followed by chemotherapy and radiotherapy.

Wagner R. *Curbside Consultation in Pediatric Ophthalmology: 49 Clinical Questions* (pp 171-173)
© 2014 SLACK Incorporated

Figure 35-1. Orbital lymph-angioma with hemorrhage.

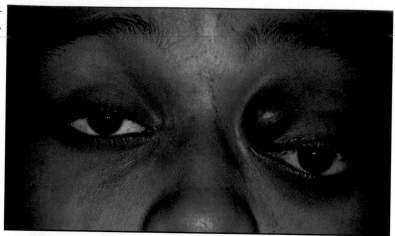

Figure 35-2. Orbitoconjunctival lymphangioma with hemorrhage.

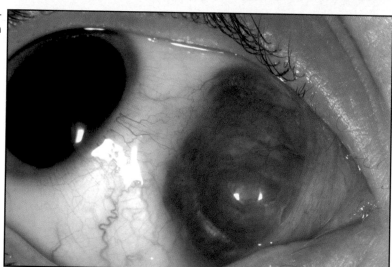

Figure 35-3. Orbital rhabdomyosarcoma.

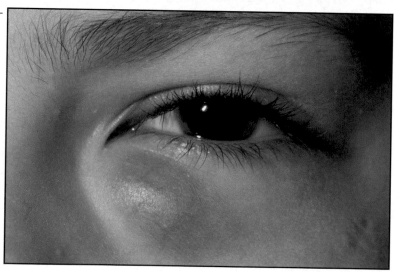

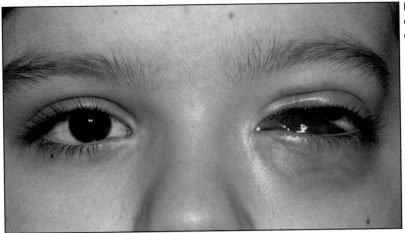

Figure 35-4. Massive orbital rhabdomyosarcoma.

Metastatic neuroblastoma to the orbit may present with proptosis and periorbital and eyelid ecchymosis. This finding can be confused with ecchymosis secondary to orbital trauma, either accidental or nonaccidental.

Suggested Readings

Shields CL, Shields JA, Honavar SG, Demerci H. The clinical spectrum of primary ophthalmic rhabdomyosarcoma. *Ophthalmol.* 2001;108:2284-2292.

Shields JA, Shields CL. *Eyelid, Conjunctival, and Orbital Tumors: An Atlas and Textbook.* 2nd ed. Philadelphia, PA: Lippincott Williams & Wilkins; 2008.

36

How Is Retinoblastoma Diagnosed? What Does the Work-up Entail, and What Measures Should I Take to Never Miss This Diagnosis?

Carol L. Shields, MD

Retinoblastoma is the most common intraocular malignancy in childhood. It is estimated that there are approximately 7000 cases per year worldwide. In the United States, it is estimated that there are approximately 350 cases per year.[1] This tumor can metastasize fairly rapidly and produce death within 1 to 2 years of detection. The most common sites for metastasis include the brain and bone marrow. Features that predict metastasis include invasive retinoblastoma into the optic nerve or choroid. Retinoblastoma can occur in one eye or (less commonly) in both eyes when there is a genetic predisposition.

Early detection of retinoblastoma is critical. The most common features include crossed eyes (strabismus) and leukocoria (white pupil). Any child with strabismus or leukocoria should be examined by an ophthalmologist. It is important to realize that any condition that results in loss of vision in a child can produce a strabismus. Wide pupillary dilation with indirect ophthalmoscopy performed by an ophthalmologist is essential to establish the diagnosis of retinoblastoma. This tumor clinically appears as a yellow-white tumor forming nodules within the retina and fed by dilated feeding vessels (Figure 36-1). As this tumor enlarges, it produces a retinal detachment and later causes glaucoma and buphthalmos (large globe). Most often retinoblastoma is detected within the first 1 to 2 years of life.

In the United States, most children are diagnosed while the tumor remains in the eye. Approximately 20% have high-risk retinoblastoma and require chemotherapy to prevent metastatic disease.[2] The most common treatments for retinoblastoma include intravenous chemotherapy for 6 months, intra-arterial chemotherapy for 6 injections, plaque radiotherapy, cryotherapy, thermotherapy, external beam radiotherapy, or enucleation. The goals of treatment are to save the patient's life and if possible, the eye and vision.

Wagner R. *Curbside Consultation in Pediatric Ophthalmology: 49 Clinical Questions* (pp 175-176) © 2014 SLACK Incorporated

Figure 36-1. Retinoblastoma.

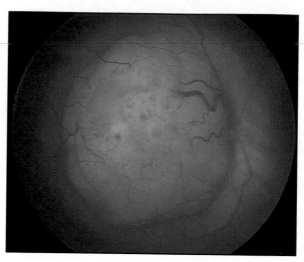

The pediatrician should be aware of retinoblastoma and should become proficient in recognizing the normal and abnormal red reflex in all infants so that this condition is not misssed. In addition, checking for abnormalities in ocular alignment ("cross eyes" or "wall eyes") is important because strabismus could be a sign of an underlying tumor.

References

1. Kivela T. The epidemiological challenge of the most frequent eye cancer: retinoblastoma, an issue of birth and death. *Br J Ophthalmol.* 2009;93:1129-1131.
2. Kaliki S, Shields CL, Rojanaporn, et al. High-risk retinoblastoma based on international classification of retinoblastoma: analysis of 519 enucleated eyes. *Ophthalmol.* 2013;120:997-1003.

Suggested Readings

Shields CL, Shields JA. Basic understanding of current classification and management of retinoblastoma. *Curr Opin Ophthalmol.* 2006;17:228-234.

Shields CL, Shields JA. Retinoblastoma management: advances in enucleation, intravenous chemoreduction, and intra-arterial chemotherapy. *Curr Opin Ophthalmol.* 2010;21:203-212.

Shields JA, Shields CL. *Intraocular Tumors: An Atlas and Textbook.* 2nd ed. Philadelphia, PA: Lippincott Williams & Wilkins; 2008.

WHAT IS THE DIFFERENTIAL DIAGNOSIS OF LEUKOCORIA?

Carol L. Shields, MD

The differential diagnosis of leukocoria (or "white pupil") includes scarred cornea, cataract, endophthalmitis (infection in the eye), retinal detachment, chorioretinal colobomas, vitreous hemorrhage, and retinoblastoma. In rare instances, if there is an ocular misalignment with the eye turned in by 15 degrees, a normal optic disc can produce leukocoria. Leukocoria basically represents reflection of a light source from the retina back to the observer. If the light is directed to the optic disc, leukocoria will be visualized. If the light is directed to normal retina, the reflex will be red. If the light is directed toward a white tumor such as retinoblastoma, the reflex will be white, as in leukocoria (Figure 37-1). Other ocular conditions can give a yellow-white reflex, including Coats' disease, vitreous hemorrhage, retinal detachment, endophthalmitis, and cataract.

Caregivers may present photographs of their child to the pediatrician showing a white pupillary reflex. All children with leukocoria should be seen by an ophthalmologist. Because of the gravity of this situation, leukocoria should prompt an urgent referral to an ophthalmologist to rule out retinoblastoma and other serious ophthalmic conditions.

Wagner R. *Curbside Consultation in Pediatric
Ophthalmology: 49 Clinical Questions* (pp 177-178)
© 2014 SLACK Incorporated

Figure 37-1. White pupil (leukocoria) in a child with retinoblastoma.

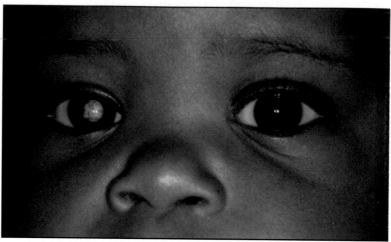

Suggested Readings

Shields CL, Schoenfeld E, Kocher K, Shukla SY, Kaliki S, Shields JA. Lesions simulating retinoblastoma (pseudoretino-blastoma) in 604 cases. *Ophthalmol.* 2013;120:311-316.

Shields CL, Shields JA. Basic understanding of current classification and management of retinoblastoma. *Curr Opin Ophthalmol.* 2006;17:228-234.

Shields CL, Shields JA. Retinoblastoma management: advances in enucleation, intravenous chemoreduction, and intra-arterial chemotherapy. *Curr Opin Ophthalmol.* 2010;21:203-212.

Shields JA, Shields CL. *Intraocular Tumors: An Atlas and Textbook.* 2nd ed. Philadelphia, PA: Lippincott Williams & Wilkins; 2008.

SECTION VIII

RETINOPATHY OF PREMATURITY

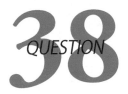

38

WHICH CHILDREN MUST BE SCREENED FOR RETINOPATHY OF PREMATURITY, AND HOW SHOULD THEY BE FOLLOWED ONCE DISCHARGED FROM THE HOSPITAL?

James Reynolds, MD

Infants who are born prematurely are at risk of developing retinopathy of prematurity (ROP), a potentially blinding disease of the retina centered on the developing vascular bed. Treatment has been available for ROP since 1988 and has been refined over the years. It currently includes peripheral retina cryoablation or laser photocoagulation and the still-controversial injection of antivascular endothelial growth factor (VEGF) in the form of bevacizumab or ranibizumab. However, to have a high success rate, treatment must be applied within a narrow window of opportunity based on retinal disease parameters. Because this is a treatable disease that is undetectable except by ophthalmologic examination, screening eye examinations become paramount.

An ROP screening protocol must answer 5 questions:

1. Who should be screened?
2. When should the initial examination be conducted?
3. How frequently should follow-up examinations be conducted?
4. When can the acute screening examinations be concluded?
5. What are the professional responsibilities of those involved?

What Are the Professional Responsibilities of Those Involved?

We can start by answering the last question first. The potential responsible parties include neonatologists, ophthalmologists, hospital administrators, nursing staff, social workers, discharge

Wagner R. *Curbside Consultation in Pediatric Ophthalmology: 49 Clinical Questions* (pp 181-185)
© 2014 SLACK Incorporated

planning staff, and community pediatricians who accept such infants into their practice. Each of these professionals will in some way be involved with ROP examinations. Clearly, they will not have equal responsibility, but each individual is an important cog in the machine. The examining ophthalmologist must be available to conduct examinations on a regular basis, be knowledgeable of ROP disease pathophysiology and disease natural history, be competent to perform examinations, and be able to treat or arrange appropriate treatment on an urgent basis. The neonatologist must also know ROP pathophysiology and natural history and must be able to order timely initial and follow-up consultations. Hospital administrators need to facilitate the institution of an appropriate screening protocol and periodically monitor that protocol. Nursing staff must be able to assist in the eye examinations, but also should participate in monitoring the timeliness of examinations per protocol and per ophthalmologist recommendation. Social workers need to educate families and improve compliance. Discharge planners need to arrange appropriate outpatient follow-up and monitor compliance in some way. Community pediatricians who accept premature infants into their practice must know the natural history of ROP, recognize the need for appropriately timed eye examinations, have arrangements with ophthalmic consultants who can provide such examinations, and monitor and improve family compliance with the necessary examinations. Some or all of these parties should establish a well-understood ROP screening protocol that specifically details the procedures that will be used and the personnel who will carry them out to ensure that all at-risk infants are examined and managed appropriately.[1]

Who Should Be Screened?

Birth weight and gestational age are not only easily determined, they are by far the most important risk factors. The incidence and severity of ROP correlates strongly with decreasing birth weight and decreasing gestational age. The multicenter ROP trials have yielded robust natural history data that have enabled the development of an evidence-based screening protocol.[2-5] However, 2 important caveats remain. For reasons of study design, the multicenter trials limited their study populations to infants with birth weights of 1250 g or less. Clearly, larger babies can also get ROP. So the inclusive screening criteria have a robust evidence-based component along with a much more empirical component that covers older, larger infants. In addition, the screening parameters used in high-wealth countries do not apply to mid-wealth countries.

All infants with birth weights of 1500 g or less or gestational ages of 30 weeks or less need an initial ophthalmologic examination. Infants qualify for examination if they fit into either category. For example, a small-for-gestational age infant with a birthweight of 1400 g but a gestational age of 32 weeks requires examination. Likewise, a 1600-g child who is 30 weeks also needs an examination. Rarely, infants that are bigger or older warrant examination if they have had an unusually challenging medical course.

When Should the Initial Examination Be Conducted?

The question of timing of the initial examination is critical. Natural history data from 2 multicenter trials—CRYO-ROP and LIGHT-ROP—were used to develop criteria based on both postmenstrual age and chronologic age of at-risk infants.[2-4] These data demonstrated an amazing fact: earlier born, younger infants developed the disease later than older infants.[2] In essence, the postmenstrual age of the infant correlated with the onset of ROP much more closely than chronologic age. The developmental maturation of the retina was a more important factor than the duration of exposure to the extrauterine environment. Hence, we developed a screening paradigm based on

Table 38-1
When to Begin Acute Retinopathy of Prematurity Screening

Gestational Age at Birth, weeks	Age at Initial Examination, weeks	
	Postmenstrual	Chronologic
22	31	9
23	31	8
24	31	7
25	31	6
26	31	5
27	31	4
28	32	4
29	33	4
30	34	4
31*	35	4
32*	36	4

* If necessary.

Adapted from Reynolds JD, Dobson V, Quinn GE, et al. Evidence-based screening criteria for retinopathy of prematurity. *Arch Ophthalmol.* 2002;120:1470-1476.

gestational age at birth. The initial examination should occur during the 1-week window in which the infant's postmenstrual age is 31 weeks or the chronologic age is 4 weeks, whichever comes later. Table 38-1 is the synthesis of this information and allows each infant's 1-week eye examination window to be readily determined at birth or upon admission to the intensive care nursery.[1]

A note of explanation is necessary to appreciate the 1-week window concept. All the large, multicenter trials used 1 week as the minimum age calculation. No infant's age was tabulated in smaller units (ie, days). Therefore, statistically, an infant who has a postmenstrual age of 31 weeks, 0 days is the same age as an infant who is 31 weeks, 6 days. They are both 31 weeks, and hence all applicable dates are counted off with 7-day/1-week increments.

How Frequently Should Follow-up Examinations Be Conducted?

We used CRYO-ROP and LIGHT-ROP data to determine who should be screened and when to initiate such screening. The ET-ROP trial provided data on the necessary frequency of examinations.[5] Although basic epidemiologic parameters determine who and when, how frequently an infant should be re-examined is a function of the observed retinal findings and the known natural

Table 38-2
Follow-up Eye Examinations Based on Retinal Findings

1 Week or Less

- Stage 1 or 2 ROP: zone I
- Stage 3 ROP: zone II
- Immature vascularization: zone I—no ROP
- Immature retina extends into posterior zone II, near the boundary of zone I
- The presence or suspected presence of aggressive posterior ROP

1 to 2 Weeks

- Immature vascularization: posterior zone II
- Stage 2 ROP: zone II
- Unequivocally regressing ROP: zone I

2 Week

- Stage 1 ROP: zone II
- Unequivocally regressing ROP: zone II
- Immature vascularization: zone II—no ROP

2 to 3 Weeks

- Stage 1 or 2 ROP: zone III
- Regressing ROP: zone III

history of disease progression, so the eye examination itself is integral to determining subsequent eye examinations. Table 38-2 lists the recommended follow-up examination intervals based on the retinal disease classification. Of course, it is imperative that such classification be accurate. We know from experience that even well-trained examiners make judgment errors in classification.[4] That is why it is so important to know the natural history of this disease so well and select a follow-up interval that is compatible with the actual examination classification and the natural history data.

When Can the Acute Screening Examinations Be Concluded?

The only remaining question is when to conclude the acute screening process (Table 38-3). Again using natural history data from the multicenter trials, we can determine when to conclude the screening based on both age and retinal findings.[2-6]

It is extremely important to note that the natural course of ROP is not limited to inpatients. Many patients will be discharged while still at risk of acute ROP. This is why social workers, discharge planners, and community pediatricians are also crucial to a successful ROP screening program. This disease plays out along a stereotyped time frame of retinal development. The maturation level of the retina in conjunction with the population epidemiology determines the progress

---

Table 38-3

When to Conclude Eye Examinations Based on Age and Retinal Findings

- Zone III retinal vascularization attained without previous zone I or II ROP (if there is examiner doubt about the zone or if the postmenstrual age is less than 35 weeks, confirmatory examinations may be warranted)
- Full retinal vascularization
- Postmenstrual age of 50 weeks and no prethreshold disease (defined as stage 3 ROP in zone II, any ROP in zone I) or worse ROP is present
- Regression of ROP (care must be taken to be sure that there is no abnormal vascular tissue present that is capable of reactivation and progression)

---

of ROP. This occurs whether the infant is an inpatient or outpatient and whether the supplemental oxygen is ongoing or concluded.

All caregivers of at-risk premature infants need to be cognizant of the possibility of ROP and the need to follow the guidelines as to whom, when, and how frequently ROP screenings are to be applied.[1]

References

1. Reynolds JD. Malpractice and the quality of care in retinopathy of prematurity (An American Ophthalmological Society Thesis). *Trans Am Ophthalmol Soc.* 2007;105:161-180.
2. Palmer EA, Flynn JT, Hardy RJ, et al. Incidence and early course of retinopathy of prematurity. *Ophthalmol.* 1991;98:1628-1640.
3. Reynolds JD, Hardy RJ, Kennedy KA, et al. Lack of efficacy of light reduction in preventing retinopathy of prematurity. *N Engl J Med.* 1998;338:1572-1576.
4. Reynolds JD, Dobson V, Quinn GE, et al. Evidence-based screening criteria for retinopathy of prematurity. *Arch Ophthalmol.* 2002;120:1470-1476.
5. Early Treatment of Retinopathy of Prematurity Cooperative Group. The incidence and course of retinopathy of prematurity: findings from the early treatment for retinopathy of prematurity study. *Pediatr.* 2005;116(1):15-23.
6. Repka MX, Palmer EA, Tung B, for the Cryotherapy for Retinopathy of Prematurity Cooperative Group. Involution of retinopathy of prematurity. *Arch Ophthalmol.* 2000;118:645-649.

Suggested Reading

Fierson WM. Policy statement: screening examination of premature infants for retinopathy of prematurity. American Academy of Pediatrics. *Pediatr.* 2013;131:189-195.

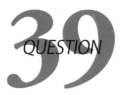

WHAT IS NEW IN THE TREATMENT OF RETINOPATHY OF PREMATURITY?

R.V. Paul Chan, MD, FACS and María Ana Martínez-Castellanos, MD

Current Treatment Options for Retinopathy of Prematurity

- Cryotherapy
- Laser photocoagulation (indirect, transscleral diode)
- Anti-vascular endothelial growth factor therapy

Despite well-defined treatment criteria, retinopathy of prematurity (ROP) continues to be a significant cause of pediatric morbidity and blindness throughout the world.[1] As a result of the findings of the CRYO-ROP (Cryotherapy for Retinopathy of Prematurity) and ET-ROP (Early Treatment for Retinopathy of Prematurity) studies, ablation of the avascular peripheral retina has been the treatment of choice for advanced disease.[2,3] Currently, treatment is recommended at type 1 prethreshold as defined by ETROP criteria. Although the outcomes after laser by ETROP criteria are improved as compared with treatment at threshold disease, the failure rate continues to be significant for posterior (zone I) disease. This poses a greater issue as increasingly younger and lower birth weight infants are able to survive. Therefore, more aggressive forms of ROP, such as aggressive posterior ROP (AP-ROP), which historically have worse functional and anatomic outcomes, may become more prevalent.[4-7]

Wagner R. *Curbside Consultation in Pediatric Ophthalmology: 49 Clinical Questions* (pp 187-192)
© 2014 SLACK Incorporated

Figure 39-1. Eye treated with ranibizumab (A) before treatment, (B) 1 week after treatment, and (C) 6 weeks after treatment.

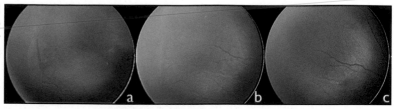

Role of Vascular Endothelial Growth Factor in Retinopathy of Prematurity

Vascular endothelial growth factor (VEGF) plays a significant role in normal vascular development and in the pathogenesis of ROP. Pathologic levels of VEGF can promote the progression of ROP with the formation of retinal and iris neovascularization.[8] Therefore, ablation of the peripheral avascular retina with cryotherapy or laser therapy may cause a reduction of VEGF levels, inducing regression of pathologic neovascularization.

Treatment Considerations

When determining what treatment to use for type-1 prethreshold ROP, several factors should be considered:

- Efficacy of the treatment
- Feasibility, ease of use, and time needed to perform the treatment
- Safety and adverse events of the treatment (systemic and local)

EFFICACY

Indirect laser photocoagulation has been the gold standard of treatment for type-1 prethreshold ROP. However, in certain situations, laser photocoagulation has not been effective (eg, zone I and AP-ROP). Unfavorable outcomes for zone I ROP after laser can be as high as approximately 30%, and it is not uncommon for AP-ROP to progress despite timely and appropriate treatment with laser.[6,7] In addition, peripheral retinal ablation for treatment-requiring ROP in zone I or posterior zone II involves destruction of a large area of avascular retina. Therefore, pharmacotherapy for ROP may help to improve outcomes in the most aggressive cases.

Pegaptanib, bevacizumab, and ranibizumab have all been reported to be effective in decreasing neovascularization associated with ROP (Figure 39-1). Intravitreal bevacizumab promotes regression of treatment-requiring ROP, and this regression often occurs quickly (Figures 39-2 and 39-3). One of the earliest reports demonstrating the use of anti-VEGF therapy for ROP was with pegaptanib. Although pegaptanib was shown to decrease vascular activity in ROP, the treatment did not prevent the retina from progressing to detachment.[9] Subsequently, a number of case series reported regression of ROP in patients treated with bevacizumab either as monotherapy or in combination with conventional laser.[10-19]

BEAT-ROP

The BEAT-ROP (Bevacizumab Eliminates the Angiogenic Threat of Retinopathy of Prematurity) study prospectively investigated the use of intravitreal bevacizumab for

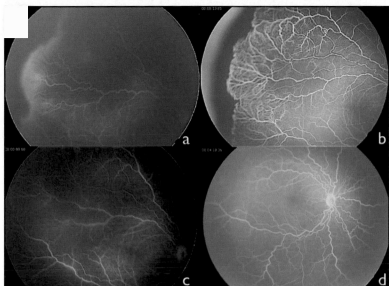

Figure 39-2. Angiogram of an eye treated for ROP with intravitreal bevacizumab as monotherapy (A) before treatment, (B) 2 weeks after treatment, (C) 6 weeks after treatment, and (D) 18 weeks after treatment.

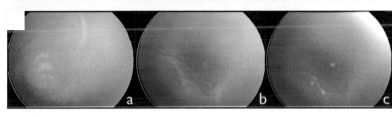

Figure 39-3. Eye treated with intravitreal bevacizumab for zone I, stage 3+ROP disease. (A) Before treatment, (B) 3 days after treatment, and (C) 16 weeks after treatment.

treatment-requiring ROP.[20] In February 2011, Mintz Hittner et al[21] presented early results from the BEAT-ROP study, which demonstrated superiority of intravitreal bevacizumab over conventional laser for zone I, stage 3+ ROP disease.

One hundred fifty study subjects were divided into 2 arms (intravitreal bevacizumab [IVB] and laser therapy). IVB was superior for zone I (p = .003) but not for posterior zone II (p = .27). Recurrence was also shown to occur later for the IVB group as compared with the laser group in both zone I and posterior zone II.

FEASIBILITY, EASE OF USE, AND TIME

Successful administration of indirect laser photocoagulation for ROP requires significant experience and skill in indirect ophthalmoscopy. Insufficient laser can lead to progression and recurrence of disease with subsequent poor outcomes. Also, in some cases, laser may require general anesthesia and can take a significant amount of time to complete.

Intravitreal anti-VEGF therapy, takes significantly less time to perform and can often be administered directly at the bedside. However, familiarity and skill with the procedure is still required. In addition, experience with indirect ophthalmoscopy is necessary for proper examination before and after the procedure to monitor for disease progression and recurrence.

SAFETY AND ADVERSE EVENTS

Although no reported systemic adverse events are associated with indirect laser photocoagulation, if general anesthesia is needed to perform laser, one must consider the risk of anesthesia for the neonate. Manipulation and pain in the nonanesthesized neonate undergoing a prolonged laser

Figure 39-4. Persistent peripheral retinal nonperfusion 9 months after IVB injection.

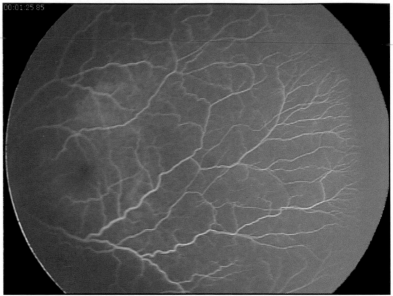

Figure 39-5. Progression of retinal detachment. (A) Before treatment and (B) 1 week after intravitreal injection of bevacizumab treatment.

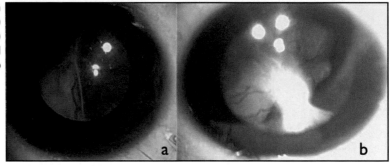

procedure may also cause significant morbidity to the child. Local adverse events may include, but are not limited to, cataract, retinal detachment, disease progression, hemorrhage, ischemia, hypotony, corneal burns, and glaucoma.

Regarding adverse events for intravitreal anti-VEGF therapy, Quiroz-Mercado et al[12] reported their results in 13 patients with ROP who were treated with IVB. Disease regression was noted in all cases, and no significant systemic adverse events have been observed in this series with 5 years of follow-up. All of the patients required only one injection of IVB to prevent progression of disease. Most patients in this cohort had some degree of myopia, and development as per the Denver Developmental Screening Test was appropriate in all but one patient.[19] Regardless of these findings, there is still significant concern that intravitreal anti-VEGF therapy for ROP may disrupt normal vascular development both locally and systemically.

Local adverse events have been reported with the use of intravitreal anti-VEGF therapy for ROP. For example, vitreous hemorrhage, prolonged peripheral retinal nonperfusion, and progression to retinal detachment have all been noted with intravitreal anti-VEGF treatment (Figures 39-4 and 39-5).[22-24]

Questions Regarding Anti-VEGF Therapy for Retinopathy of Prematurity

It has been suggested that "intravitreal bevacizumab should become the treatment of choice for zone I retinopathy of prematurity."[25] However, timing and number of injections, injection technique, choice of drug, drug dosage, and required follow-up schedule after injection are among the many questions that still remain in using anti-VEGF agents for ROP.

Conclusion

Over the past several decades, our armamentarium for the treatment of ROP has expanded from cryotherapy to laser and now to intravitreal anti-VEGF therapy. Laser photocoagulation has been very effective in managing patients with type-1 prethreshold without direct systemic adverse events. However, peripheral ablation may promote local adverse events and if general anesthesia is required, the child may be at risk for significant morbidity. Currently, we have learned that intravitreal anti-VEGF therapy is effective in promoting regression of ROP and we know the short-term outcomes of this treatment modality. Anti-VEGF therapy works well for zone I, stage 3+ disease. However, it is still too early to claim that anti-VEGF therapy is the standard of care for all types of treatment requiring ROP. The long term safety of anti-VEGF therapy has not been determined in a large, multicenter prospective trial, and given the fact that conventional laser for type-1 prethreshold ROP is a proven method of treatment, we cannot exclude laser from our treatment paradigm.

References

1. Flynn JT, Bancalari E, Bachynski BN, et al. Retinopathy of prematurity. Diagnosis, severity, and natural history. *Ophthalmol.* 1987;94(6):620-629.
2. Multicenter trial of cryotherapy for retinopathy of prematurity. Preliminary results. Cryotherapy for Retinopathy of Prematurity Cooperative Group. *Arch Ophthalmol.* 1988;106(4):471-479.
3. Early Treatment for Retinopathy of Prematurity Cooperative Group. Revised indications for the treatment of retinopathy of prematurity: results of the Early Treatment for Retinopathy of Prematurity randomized trial. *Arch Opthalmol.* 2003;121(12):1684-1694.
4. The Committee for the Classification of Retinopathy of Prematurity. An international classification of retinopathy of prematurity. *Arch Ophthalmol.* 1984;102(8):1130-1134.
5. International Committee for the Classification of Retinopathy of Prematurity. The International Classification of Retinopathy of Prematurity revisited. *Arch Ophthalmol.* 2005;123(7):991-999.
6. Drenser KA, Trese MT, Capone A Jr. Aggressive posterior retinopathy of prematurity. *Retina.* 2010;30(4):S37-S40.
7. Kychenthal A, Dorta P, Katz X. Zone I retinopathy of prematurity: clinical characteristics and treatment outcomes. *Retina.* 2006;26(7):S11-S15.
8. Pierce EA, Foley ED, Smith LE. Regulation of vascular endothelial growth factor by oxygen in a model of retinopathy of prematurity. *Arch Ophthalmol.* 1996;114(10):1219-1228.
9. Trese MT, Capone A Jr, Drenser K. Macugen in retinopathy of prematurity. *Invest Ophthalmol Vis Sci.* 2006;47:2330.
10. Chung EJ, Kim JH, Ahn HS, Koh HJ. Combination of laser photocoagulation and intravitreal bevacizumab (Avastin) for aggressive zone I retinopathy of prematurity. *Graefes Arch Clin Exp Ophthalmol.* 2007;245(11):1727-1730.
11. Mintz-Hittner HA, Kuffel RR. Intravitreal injection of bevacizumab (Avastin) for treatment of stage 3 retinopathy of prematurity in zone I or posterior zone II. *Retina.* 2008;28(6):831-838.
12. Quiroz-Mercado H, Martinez-Castellanos MA, Hernandez-Rojas ML, Salazar-Teran N, Chan RVP. Antiangiogenic therapy with intravitreal bevacizumab for retinopathy of prematurity. *Retina.* 2008;28(3):S19-S25.
13. Lalwani GA, Berrocal AM, Murray TG, et al. Off-label use of intravitreal bevacizumab (Avastin) for salvage treatment in progressive threshold retinopathy of prematurity. *Retina.* 2008; 28(3):S13-S18.

14. Micieli JA, Surkont M, Smith AF. A systematic analysis of the off-label use of bevacizumab for severe retinopathy of prematurity. *Am J Ophthalmol.* 2009;148(4):536-543.

15. Shah PK, Narendran V, Tawansy KA, et al. Intravitreal bevacizumab (Avastin) for post laser anterior segment ischemia in aggressive posterior retinopathy of prematurity. *Indian J Ophthalmol.* 2007;55(1):75-76.

16. Travassos A, Teixeira S, Ferreira P, et al. Intravitreal bevacizumab in aggressive posterior retinopathy of prematurity. *Ophthalmic Surg Lasers Imaging.* 2007;38(3):233-237.

17. Wu WC, Yeh PT, Chen SN, Yang CM, Lai CC, Kuo HK. Effects and complications of bevacizumab use in patients with retinopathy of prematurity: a multicenter study in Taiwan. *Ophthalmol.* 2011;118(1):176-183.

18. Kusaka S, Shima C, Wada K, et al. Efficacy of intravitreal injection of bevacizumab for severe retinopathy of prematurity: a pilot study. *Br J Ophthalmol.* 2008;92(11):1450-1455.

19. Guerrero-Naranjo JL, Martinez-Castellanos MA, Morales-Canton V, Garcia-Aguirre G, Chan P, Quiroz-Mercado H. Five years follow up of intravitreal bevacizumab therapy in the treatment of retinopathy of prematurity. Anatomical, functional, and neurodevelopmental analysis. Paper presented at: The Association for Research in Vision and Ophthalmology Annual Meeting; April 22, 2011; Fort Lauderdale, FL.

20. ClinicalTrials.gov. *Bevacizumab eliminates the angiogenic threat of retinopathy of prematurity (BEAT-ROP).* http://clinicaltrials.gov/ct2/show/NCT00622726. Accessed June 21, 2011.

21. Mintz-Hittner HA, Kennedy KA, Chuang AZ; BEAT-ROP Cooperative Group. Efficacy of intravitreal bevacizumab for stage 3+ retinopathy of prematurity. *N Engl J Med.* 2011;364(7):603-615.

22. Honda S, Hirabayashi H, Tsukahara Y, Negi A. Acute contraction of the proliferative membrane after an intravitreal injection of bevacizumab for advanced retinopathy of prematurity. *Graefes Arch Clin Exp Ophthalmol.* 2008;246(7):1061-1063.

23. Rodriguez Torres EO, Martinez MA, Quiroz Mercado H, et al. Worldwide experiences with intravitreal anti-VEGFs for ROP. Paper presented at: The Association for Research in Vision and Ophthalmology Annual Meeting; April 22, 2011; Fort Lauderdale, FL.

24. Martinez-Castellanos MA, Morales-Canton V, Saravia MJ, Chan RV, Quiroz-Mercado H. Variations in the morphology of the retinal vessels following intravitreal anti-VEGF therapy for treatment requiring retinopathy of prematurity. Paper presented at: The Association for Research in Vision and Ophthalmology Annual Meeting; April 22, 2011; Fort Lauderdale, FL.

25. Reynolds JD. Bevacizumab for retinopathy of prematurity. *N Engl J Med.* 2011;364(7):677-678.

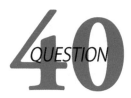

QUESTION 40

WHY DOES MYOPIA OCCUR FREQUENTLY IN CHILDREN WITH SIGNIFICANT RETINOPATHY OF PREMATURITY?

Rudolph S. Wagner, MD

It is common for children who were premature at birth and had retinopathy of prematurity (ROP) to require glasses for correction of myopia at an early age. The myopia is often significant and in the range of what is considered high myopia (> -5.00 diopters). Furthermore, many of these children will require occlusion therapy to treat refractive amblyopia resulting from asymmetric myopia. The myopia associated with ROP is generally not the axial type of myopia seen in typical progressive myopia of childhood.

Myopia in Retinopathy of Prematurity

ROP remains one of the leading causes of childhood blindness worldwide. The disease process can result in loss of vision due to retinal detachment, poor macular development, and anterior segment ischemia. The finding of a thicker macula in ROP may also result in poor vision. This could be due to disruption of lateral migration of inner retinal cells during normal development of the fovea. It can also result in other ocular disorders such as refractive error, amblyopia, strabisumus, cataracts, and glaucoma. It is extremely frustrating when poor vision from high myopia or refractive amblyopia follows therapy that halts the progression of ROP. Myopia often develops within the first 6 to 9 months of life in ROP patients, particularly in those with more severe disease and following treatment. High myopia and anisometropia present major obstacles to achieving satisfactory vision in these children. Cryotherapy and laser ablation of peripheral retinal neovascularization have been used to treat ROP, with favorable outcomes. However, substantial myopia is frequently found in patients treated with either cryotherapy or laser photocoagulation. Recently, intravitreal bevacizumab, an antibody against vascular endothelial growth factor (VEGF) has

Wagner R. *Curbside Consultation in Pediatric Ophthalmology: 49 Clinical Questions* (pp 193-196)
© 2014 SLACK Incorporated

been shown to have significant benefits for stage 3+ ROP in zone I when compared with conventional laser therapy and may reduce the incidence of myopia after treatment.

Myopia is of significant concern in infants with ROP. The prevalence of myopia in premature children is negatively correlated with birth weight and gestational age and positively correlated with greater severity of ROP. The exact cause of myopia in premature infants has not been determined, but many studies have been conducted to correlate ocular measurements with the degree of myopia, and increased lens thickness has consistently been found to be associated with ROP. In preterm infants with ROP, the main mechanism of myopia is greater lens thickness, whereas preterm infants without ROP develop myopia due to increased axial length, similar to the progressive myopia we see in many older children. It is likely that an optical component in the anterior segment (such as anterior chamber depth or lens thickness), not axial length, causes the high refractive error in patients with threshold retinopathy.

Possible Mechanisms in the Development of Myopia

Several theories have been proposed to explain the etiology of myopia in premature and ROP patients. In normal development, full-term infants become slightly hyperopic in the first few years of life due to a process called *emmetropization*, in which a reduction in corneal curvature and lens power balances an increasing vitreous cavity length. In low birth weight preterm infants, disruption of this process, such as by earlier exposure to light and visual images, may result in a slight reduction of hyperopia. However, in preterm infants with ROP, the disruption of emmetropization results in significant myopia, indicating that additional mechanisms are likely present. It is postulated that the mechanism of myopia in preterm infants with ROP is due to the embryologic derivation of both the peripheral retina and lens zonules from the neuroectoderm. Because ROP affects the peripheral retina, impaired development of lens zonules may also occur. This results in decreased tension on the lens and therefore increased lens thickness and subsequent myopia.

Treatment of Retinopathy of Prematurity and Myopia Development

Treatment of ROP may also influence myopia. The CRYO-ROP study compared myopia between cryotherapy-treated patients and controls and found a higher incidence of myopia >8 diopters in the treated group, possibly indicating that increased myopia was due to cryotherapy treatment. Some argue that because the severity of ROP is correlated with the degree of myopia, the eyes that receive treatment are those with more severe disease and therefore will inherently develop greater refractive error. However, the refractive outcome at 10 years of patients with threshold ROP treated with laser photocoagulation or cryotherapy found that eyes treated with cryotherapy were significantly more myopic than those treated with laser (SE -7.65 D versus -4.48 D; P = .019). Various factors to establish the cause of myopia have been investigated and no statistical difference in anterior corneal curvature or central corneal thickness between the 2 treatment groups was found. The cryotherapy-treated eyes had a significantly shallower anterior chamber and thicker lens compared with laser treatment. In groups that received both therapies, the crystalline lens power was most strongly correlated to refractive outcome. Therefore, the degree of myopia is not only affected by severity of disease, but also by treatment modality.

Preliminary evidence indicates that babies treated with bevacizumb intravitreal injection may be less likely to develop myopia. The difference in refractive outcome between cryotherapy, laser treatment, and bevacizumab may be due to the destruction of the peripheral retina in cryotherapy and laser ablation. Tissue destruction may result in abnormal maturation of the zonules, ciliary body, or lens. Reduced tension causes myopia and increased lens thickness, which was consistently noted. Cryotherapy inflicts more severe damage to the retina, resulting in greater myopia compared with laser-treated patients. Bevacizumab treatment does not inflict direct tissue destruction of the peripheral retina, and therefore is less likely to interfere with development of the zonules and lens. The peripheral retinal vessels continued to develop with intravitreal bevacizumab treatment, whereas laser resulted in permanent damage of the peripheral tissue.

The time course for the development of myopia can be important to predict the effectiveness of various treatments. Quinn et al looked at the prevalence of myopia between 3 months and 5.5 years of age in preterm infants with and without ROP and found that the presence of myopia at 3 months is most predictive of whether myopia will be present in the future. They found that in patients with severe acute phase ROP, the proportion of eyes with high myopia (>=5 D) doubled between 3 months and 1 year but was steady thereafter until at least 5.5 years. There was no change in proportion of myopia from birth to 3 months to 5.5 years in patients with no or only mild ROP.

Quinn et al also evaluated visual function outcomes of patients enrolled in the Early Treatment of Retinopathy of Prematurity (ET-ROP) study at 3 years of age to determine if development of myopia or high myopia was related to early treatment at prethreshold disease, or conventional management that initiated when ROP reached threshold. They found no treatment-related difference in the prevalence of myopia as the spherical equivalent of the refractive error was greater than or equal to 0.25 D at 3 years. They found that the prevalence of myopia increases between 6 and 9 months, but no further significant increase is noted between 9 months and 3 years. This time course is also consistent with previous findings from the CRYO-ROP study.

Therefore, if a patient does not show myopia within the first year of life, development of myopia in the future is unlikely unless there are genetic factors predisposing to progressive myopia. Worsening of refractive error in previously mentioned studies was only a change in distribution of the myopia to a more severe error, not a change in prevalence.

Although bevacizumab and other VEGF inhibitors display many advantages over cryotherapy and laser ablation for ROP, there are some concerns with its use. First, the long-term efficacy is not established. In a retrospective review of 9 patients conducted by Hu et al, late reactivation and progression of ROP was shown at an average of 49.3 weeks postmenstrual age and an average of 14.4 weeks after initial treatment. Five of the 9 patients had stage 5 retinal detachment. However, no eyes that received laser treatment had recurrence or progression to retinal detachment. This may be due to bevacizumab's transient effect on VEGF, whereas laser ablation creates a permanent change on the retina. In addition, the epithelial adhesions from laser treatment may make it less likely that the retina detaches in laser-treated eyes compared with an intravitreal injection of bevacizumab. Recurrent disease was shown to be most favorably treated with laser therapy.

Lastly, another concern with the use of bevacizumab is the possibility of absorption from the vitreous cavity into systemic circulation, thereby affecting the levels of VEGF throughout the body. The effects of depressed VEGF concentrations in systemic circulation of infants is still unknown. Sato et al measured the serum concentrations of bevacizumab and VEGF before and 1 day, 1 week, and 2 weeks after intravitreal injection of 0.25 mg and 0.5 mg of bevacizumab. They reported a significant negative correlation between serum bevacizumab and VEGF with the injections. This raises a concern for the systemic effect of an anti-VEGF antibody in the circulation of a premature child.

Conclusion

It should come as no surprise that many of your patients who had ROP will have reduced acuity and require glasses. It is important that these children have frequent screenings for visual acuity and receive regular ophthalmologic care.

Acknowledgments

I would like to thank Lekha Ravindraraj, MD, for her assistance in researching and contributing to this chapter.

Suggested Readings

Beri S, Malhotra M, Dhawan A, et al. A neuroectodermal hypothesis of the cause and relationship of myopia in retinopathy of prematurity. *J Pediatr Ophthalmol Strabismus*. 2009;46:146-150.

Garcia-Valenzuela E, Kaufman LM. High myopia associated with retinopathy of prematurity is primarily lenticular. *J AAPOS*. 2005;9:121-128.

Graham E, Quinn GE, Dobson V, et al. Progression of myopia and high myopia in the early treatment for retinopathy of prematurity study: findings to 3 years of age. *Ophthalmol*. 2008;115:1058-1064.

Harder BC, von Baltz S, Schlichtenbrede FC, et al. Early refractive outcome after intravitreous bevacizumab for retinopathy of prematurity. *Arch Ophthalmol*. 2012;130:800-801.

Hu J, Blair MP, Shapiro MJ, et al. Reactivation of retinopathy of prematurity after bevacizumab injection. *Arch Ophthalmol*. 2012;130(8):1000-1006

McLoone EM, O'Keefe M, McLoone SF. Long-term refractive and biometric outcomes following diode laser therapy for retinopathy of prematurity. *J AAPOS*. 2006;10:454-459.

Mintz-Hittner HA, Kennedy KA, Chuang AZ, et al. Efficacy of intravitreal bevacizumab for stage 3+ retinopathy of prematurity. *N Engl J Med*. 2011;364:603-615.

Sato T, Wada K, Arahori H, et al. Serum concentrations of bevacizumab (avastin) and vascular endothelial growth factor in infants with retinopathy of prematurity. *Am J Ophthalmol*. 2012;153:327-333.

SECTION IX

TEARING AND
EYELID DISORDERS

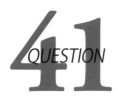

MY NEW PATIENT IS HAVING A PROBLEM WITH TEARING. HOW CAN I HELP HIM?

Linda Nakanishi, MD

Many factors may contribute to tearing in a child, so a thorough history is helpful. For tearing that begins shortly after birth, the differential diagnosis includes ophthalmia neonatorum, congenital glaucoma, nasolacrimal duct obstruction, birth trauma, and eyelid malformation. For tearing that begins a little later in childhood, ask about allergies, medical conditions, medications, and ocular injuries. To help narrow down your list of possible diagnoses, find out when the tearing occurs. In an allergic child, tearing may occur after outdoor play or contact with pets. Tearing may also occur after using a new soap, shampoo, or lotion. When a child has a cold, the nasal mucosa may swell, block the nasolacrimal duct, and lead to tearing. A patient with a cold may also tear secondary to infection or inflammation of the eyes. Next, find out about chronic medical conditions as well as routine medications. Conditions such as juvenile rheumatoid arthritis, AIDS, or thyroid disease may predispose the patient to dry eyes and secondary tearing. Similarly, medications that treat chronic conditions such as allergies may cause dryness of the child's eyes and subsequent tearing. Consider trauma as a cause of tearing. A child may be tearing due to damage to the eye and nasolacrimal drainage system. Once you have completed the history, you are ready to examine the patient.

What Eyelid Problems Are Associated With Tearing?

CRANIAL NERVE VII PALSY (BELL'S PALSY)

A patient with a cranial nerve VII palsy will tear because the eye is dry and irritated. The eye becomes dry because the eyelids do not close all the way during a blink or when the child is sleeping. When evaluating Bell's palsy, have the patient squeeze his or her eyes shut. The side with the

Wagner R. *Curbside Consultation in Pediatric*
Ophthalmology: 49 Clinical Questions (pp 199-202)
© 2014 SLACK Incorporated

Bell's palsy may not close all the way. If the eyelids close all the way, try to gently open both eyes. The eyelids on the side with the Bell's palsy will be easier to open. You may instill fluorescein dye and examine the eye with a blue filter on a pen light. The eye with the palsy will stain due to dryness. Treatment of Bell's palsy includes artificial tears and ointment. In more severe cases, have the parent tape the eyelids closed when the child is sleeping. If the Bell's palsy does not resolve and the child has a severe dry eye, refer him or her for a gold weight implant in the upper eyelid. The gold weight helps the eyelid close fully over the front of the eye during a blink and keeps the eyelids closed at night.

EYELID COLOBOMA

Does your patient have tearing and a missing segment of eyelid? This may indicate an eyelid coloboma. Treat the eye with lubricating eye ointment aggressively until the coloboma can be surgically repaired.[1]

CHALAZION

Is the tearing accompanied by a bump on the eyelid? A chalazion forms when an eyelid gland becomes plugged. A chalazion may increase in size and cause irritation and tearing. Treatment includes warm compresses 4 times a day until the chalazion drains. A chalazion that is unresponsive to conservative treatment may be incised and drained. If there is a secondary conjunctivitis, consider prescribing a topical ophthalmic antibiotic. A coexisting eyelid infection requires oral antibiotics.

ENTROPION

Is the patient's eyelid sitting in the correct position? If the eyelids are turning in toward the globe, he or she has an entropion. Patients with an entropion develop ocular irritation and tearing because the eyelashes rub the front of the eye. Treatment includes aggressive lubrication of the eye and referral for surgical repair.

EPIBLEPHARON

A patient born with an extra fold of tissue in the lower eyelid has an epiblepharon. This fold of tissue causes the lower eyelid to turn inward. The eyelashes contact the front of the eye and cause irritation and tearing. As the child's face matures, the eyelid position changes so that the lashes no longer contact the globe. Initial therapy includes artificial tear drops and lubricating eye ointment. If the epiblepharon does not resolve with facial maturation, refer for surgery to remove the fold.[1]

PRESEPTAL AND ORBITAL CELLULITIS

Is the tearing accompanied by red and swollen eyelids? When you examine the patient, ask the patient to move his or her eyes in all directions. A patient with full extraocular rotations is likely to have a preseptal cellulitis. If the patient cannot move his or her eyes in all directions, this indicates an orbital cellulitis. Young patients with cellulitis are typically admitted to the hospital and placed on intravenous antibiotics.

NASOLACRIMAL DUCT OBSTRUCTION

Is there discharge at the puncta in an otherwise white and quiet eye? This child likely has a nasolacrimal duct obstruction. The child may respond to Krigler massage with topical antibiotics as needed. If the patient continues to tear and has discharge after conservative therapy, refer to an ophthalmologist for nasolacrimal duct probing. Nasolacrimal duct probing is successful in approximately 70% to 97% of patients.[2,3]

What Problems of the Conjunctiva Are Associated With Tearing?

CONJUNCTIVAL FOREIGN BODY

The conjunctiva covers the white of the eye and the inside of the eyelids. Look for a foreign body on the globe or lodged underneath the eyelid. For superficial foreign bodies, numb the eye with proparacaine eye drops and gently remove the material with a cotton-tipped applicator.

CONJUNCTIVITIS

CONTACT LENS—RELATED CONJUNCTIVITIS (GIANT PAPILLARY CONJUNCTIVITIS)

If your patient wears contact lenses, he or she may have bumps on the underside of the eyelids called giant papillae. These giant papillae irritate the eye and cause tearing. This condition also makes it difficult to wear contact lenses. Treatment includes switching from extended wear contact lenses to daily-wear lenses. It may also include switching from soft to hard contact lenses. In severe cases, the contact lenses may be discontinued.

CHEMICAL CONJUNCTIVITIS

In a newborn presenting with red and tearing eyes within 24 hours after birth, consider a chemical conjunctivitis. The baby's eyes may be reacting to the topical drop (silver nitrate, povidine iodine, antibiotic drop) that is given as prophylaxis against eye infection.[4]

INFECTIOUS CONJUNCTIVITIS (OPHTHALMIA NEONATORUM)

In an infant with tearing and discharge, take eye cultures to look for infections such as gonorrhea and chlamydia. A patient with a gonorrhea infection of the eye needs a rigorous regimen of antibiotics to avoid rapid perforation of the eye. A child with a chronic conjunctivitis due to chlamydia requires topical ocular and oral medications to treat possible coexisting systemic problems.

ALLERGIC CONJUNCTIVITIS

A child may tear because he or she suffers from allergies. The underside of his or her eyelids may have bumps on them called follicles. Treatment of allergic conjunctivitis includes oral allergy medications as well as topical allergy and anti-inflammatory eye drops.

What Cornea Problems Cause Tearing?

CORNEAL FOREIGN BODY AND CORNEAL ABRASION

The cornea is the clear tissue at the front of the eye. In a patient who complains of foreign body sensation, use a pen light or direct ophthalmoscope and take a look at the eye. If there is a corneal foreign body, it needs to be removed. Some ophthalmologists use a diamond burr, while others use a 25-gauge needle at the slit lamp to remove the foreign body. The resulting corneal abrasion is treated with an antibiotic drop or ointment.

CORNEAL DERMOID

Is there a bump bridging the inferotemporal cornea and conjunctiva? This may be a corneal dermoid. Sometimes the dermoid can cause poor lubrication of the adjacent cornea with ocular irritation and tearing. If the dermoid is large and the adjacent cornea stains with fluorescein dye, refer for further evaluation.

CORNEAL INFECTION

Infection of the cornea causes tearing. If the child's eye stains with fluorescein dye in a branching pattern, consider infection with a herpes virus. If the patient has an ulcer on the cornea, refer him or her to an ophthalmologist for eye cultures and treatment.

CONGENITAL GLAUCOMA

A child with congenital glaucoma may present with tearing, corneal clouding, and light sensitivity. As part of your evaluation, you may try to measure the horizontal corneal diameter by placing a paper ruler across the patient's forehead. If the horizontal corneal diameter is greater than 12 mm, consider infantile or juvenile glaucoma. If possible, check the patient's eye pressures with a tonometer. Timely referral to an ophthalmologist for intraocular pressure evaluation and treatment is the next step.[5]

What Anterior Chamber Problems Are Associated With Tearing?

When a child develops intraocular inflammation from trauma, infection, or autoimmune diseases (juvenile idiopathic arthritis,[6] sarcoidosis), he or she may present with tearing and photophobia. A team of specialists will be needed to treat the systemic and ocular problems of this child. Treatment of the intraocular inflammation typically requires dilating and anti-inflammatory drops several times a day.

References

1. Katowitz WR, Katowitz JA. Congenital and developmental eyelid abnormalities. *Plast Reconstr Surg.* 2009;124S:93e-105e.
2. Pediatric Eye Disease Investigator Group. Primary treatment of nasolacrimal duct obstruction with nasolacrimal duct intubation in children younger than 4 years of age. *J AAPOS.* 2008;12:445-450.
3. Takahashi Y, Kakizaki H, Chan WO, Selva D. Management of congenital nasolacrimal duct obstruction. *Acta Ophthalmol.* 2010;88:506-513.
4. Isenberg SJ, Apt L, Del Signore M, et al. A double application approach to ophthalmia neonatorum prophylaxis. *Br J Ophthalmol.* 2003;87:1449-1452.
5. Ho CL, Walton DS. Primary congenital glaucoma: 2004 update. *J Pediatr Ophthalmol Strabismus.* 2004;41(5):271-288.
6. Sabri K, Saurenmann RK, Silerman ED, Levin AV. Course, complications and outcome of juvenile arthritis-related uveitis. *J AAPOS.* 2008;12:539-545.

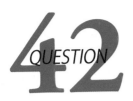

WHAT IS NASOLACRIMAL DUCT OBSTRUCTION?
HOW IS IT MANAGED?
WHEN SHOULD I REFER THESE CHILDREN?

Suqin Guo, MD and Nina Ni, MD

What Is Nasolacrimal Duct Obstruction?

Approximately 5% of infants suffer from nasolacrimal duct obstruction (NLDO). This is a congenital blockage of the tear drainage system. Common causes of NLDO include narrowing of the duct or the presence of an abnormal membrane located at the nasal (distal) end of the nasolacrimal duct within the nasal cavity. Symptoms are typically seen at 1 to 2 months of age in most (80% to 90%) infants with the condition. Because many infants produce tears at a greater rate after the first few months of life, the signs and symptoms often increase over time although the obstruction is present at birth.

Infants present with excessive tearing (epiphora) or wet-looking eyes with mucous discharge. Other clinical signs include redness and swelling of the lower eyelids. Associated infections are common (Figure 42-1). If the infection is not treated promptly, dacryocystitis or orbital cellulitis may develop, both of which could cause severe visual damage requiring intravenous antibiotics and inpatient care. A culture of the discharge often yields multiple bacterial species. The retention of dye after instillation of fluorescein dye solution to the involved eye can help to confirm the diagnosis of NLDO.

Differential diagnosis includes blepharoconjunctivitis and mucocele of the lacrimal sac. Other causes of excessive tearing are occasionally confused with NLDO; these include corneal edema, anterior uveitis, and congenital glaucoma.

Wagner R. *Curbside Consultation in Pediatric
Ophthalmology: 49 Clinical Questions* (pp 203-205)
© 2014 SLACK Incorporated

Figure 42-1. A child with NLDO showing mild infection of the lower eyelids in both eyes.

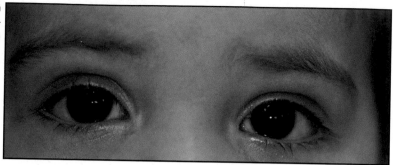

How Is It Managed?

NONSURGICAL TREATMENT

Conservative management can be initiated with digital massage of the nasolacrimal sac. It is performed by placing a fingertip to the inner corner of the eye and pressing downward slowly several times daily. This type of massage may drain the mucus in the lacrimal sac and induce hydrostatic pressure on the obstruction. If there is secondary infection, broad-spectrum topical antibiotics should be used. Systemic antibiotics are often needed to treat secondary dacryocystitis and orbital cellulitis. The latter may also require orbital imaging (computed tomography [CT] scan or magnetic resonance imaging [MRI]) to rule out an orbital abscess, which could require surgical intervention.

SURGICAL TREATMENT

Over 70% to 80% of NLDOs resolve spontaneously by 12 months of age with nonsurgical treatment. If NLDO does not resolve by 12 months of age, spontaneous resolution would be unlikely, and probing of the nasolacrimal duct is needed.[1,2]

Probing of the nasolacrimal duct is often used as the first surgical option. A Bowman probe (wire) is inserted via the upper and lower lacrimal puncta and advanced through the lacrimal sac and duct, exiting at the inferior meatus below the inferior turbinate of the nose. There is often a greater than 90% success rate with initial probing, given that it is performed properly. Repeated probing may be necessary if the first procedure fails.

Balloon dilation of the nasolacrimal duct is a popular adjunctive technique to probing for blockage associated with scarring or constriction of the nasolacrimal duct. An inflatable balloon, integrated into the tip of a wire probe, is inserted and advanced into the nasolacrimal duct system. This technique has been successful for dilating the tear drainage system. In recent years, more and more surgeons are using balloon dilation and probing as the initial surgical procedure.

Intubation of the nasolacrimal duct is recommended when repeated (more than 2 or 3) probing and ballooning dilation procedures fail. Silicone tubing is inserted through the upper and/or lower lacrimal puncta, advanced along the lacrimal sac and duct, and then passed into the nose. The silicone tubing is kept in the nasolacrimal duct system for a few months. Both monocanicular and bicanicular tubes are available for use.

DACRYOCYSTOCELE

Dacryocystocele is a rare form of NLDO. It is a result of obstruction both distally at the Hasner valve and proximally at the Rosenmuller valve within the nasolacrimal duct system. The clinical presentation is a bluish and tender swelling nasal to the medial canthus (over the nasolacrimal sac).

Differential diagnosis is critical, and orbital imaging can be useful because these lesions may appear similar to epidermal dermoid cysts, periocular hemangiomas, and meningoencephaloceles. Referral to an ophthalmologist for diagnostic confirmation and further management is often warranted. Some characteristic radiologic features of these lesions include bone changes on CT scan for orbital dermoid cysts and irregular acoustic ultrasound features with high flow pattern in infantile hemangiomas. Also of note, biopsy of a meningoencephalocele should be avoided because it can lead to cerebrospinal fluid leakage and increase the risk of meningitis.

Once a diagnosis has been established, noninvasive medical approaches are commonly used as initial treatments for an uninfected dacryocystocele. These include a combination of systemic and local broad-spectrum antibiotics, warm compresses, and nasolacrimal sac massage. Application of digital massage on the lacrimal sac serves to decompress and drain the dacryocystocele. Intranasal surgery may be indicated if the cystocele leads to respiratory distress. Lacrimal probing or ballooning is indicated in the event of dacryocystitis, orbital cellulitis, and nonresolution of the cystocele after nonsurgical treatment. Some authors recommend early probing to minimize the risk of developing dacryocystitis. Once infected, however, incisional drainage of the dacryocystocele through the skin should be avoided due to the risk of persistent fistula track formation.

When Should I Refer These Children?

If a child presents with any of the following conditions/complications, referral to an ophthalmologist or pediatric ophthalmologist should be made promptly for proper treatment:

- Infection associated with NLDO, including discharge and swelling of the eyelids
- Resistance to topical antibiotic treatment
- Associated severe blepharoconjunctivitis, dacryocystocele, dacryocystitis, or orbital cellulitis

References

1. Pediatric Eye Disease Investigator Group. Resolution of congenital nasolacrimal duct obstruction with nonsurgical management. *Arch Ophthalmol.* 2012;130(6):730-734.
2. MacEwen CJ, Young JD. Epiphora during the first year of life. *Eye.* 1991;5(Pt 5):596-600.

Suggested Readings

Becker BB. The treatment of congenital dacryocystocele. *Am J Ophthalmol.* 2006;142:835-838.

Calhoun JH. Problems of the lacrimal system in children. *Pediatr Clin North Am.* 1987;34(6):1457-1465.

Guo S, Olitsky SE, Weaver DT. Management of a nasolacrimal duct fistula. *J Pediatr Ophthalmol Strabismus.* 2013;50(3):136-137.

Raab EL. The lacrimal drainage system. In: American Academy of Ophthalmology, Basic and Clinical Sciences Course. Section 6: Pediatric Ophthalmology and Strabismus. San Francisco, CA: AAO; 2010-2011:203-206.

Shields JA, Shields CL. Orbital cysts of childhood: classification, clinical features, and management. *Surv Ophthalmol.* 2004;49:281-299.

HOW DOES A CONGENITAL DACRYOCELE PRESENT, AND HOW SHOULD I MANAGE THESE INFANTS?

Rudolph S. Wagner, MD

A likely occurrence is that you encounter a newborn infant either in the nursery or in your office shortly after birth with a firm, bluish-colored mass displacing the medial lower eyelid upward (Figure 43-1). There is a mucous discharge coming from the eye but there is no conjunctival vascular injection. In other words, the typical signs of a red eye are not present. The mother may observe the baby having difficulty breathing while breast feeding. This may indicate that an intranasal mucocele is present.

Clinical Characteristics

Also known as lacrimal sac mucocele, dacryocystocele, or amniotocele, a dacryocele is cystic distension of the lacrimal sac manifesting in the perinatal period. The clinical appearance is a tense bluish swelling just below the medial canthal area that displaces the medial lower eyelid superiorly. Dacryoceles are more common in female infants, are mostly unilateral, and are successfully treated without the need for general anesthesia in about 50% of cases. These infants are treated with systemic antibiotics and warm compresses. These may occur bilaterally and distort the facial appearance of the infant. They may be present at birth and can be detected by prenatal ultrasound in some cases. Dacryoceles are usually discovered in the nursery but may not be recognized until the baby leaves the hospital because mucous accumulates in the lacrimal sac. The palpable mass is firm, unmoveable, and sometimes tender. With firm digital massage of the lacrimal sac, decompression of the mass may occur, sometimes suddenly, with mucoid discharge expressed from the puncta and/or the nasal cavity (Figure 43-2). The cyst may reform following digital massage if the proximal and distal obstruction of the lacrimal sac remains as mucous accumulates again. In

Wagner R. *Curbside Consultation in Pediatric*
Ophthalmology: 49 Clinical Questions (pp 207-209)
© 2014 SLACK Incorporated

Figure 43-1. Dacryocele with a characteristic bluish subcutaneous mass displacing the left medial lower eyelid superiorly.

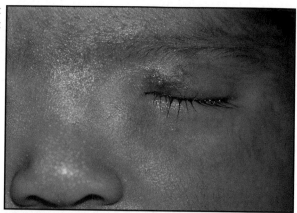

Figure 43-2. Reflux of mucus from the superior and inferior puncta during digital massage of a congenital dacryocele.

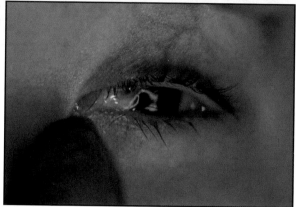

some cases, bacteria may enter the distended sac and an acute, painful dacryocystitis may occur. The findings of a tender fluctuant mass in the area of the lacrimal sac in a febrile infant are suggestive of an infection. Acute dacryocystitis may result in preseptal, or in some cases postseptal, orbital cellulitis and must be treated aggressively with systemic antibiotics and warm compresses.

Infants are obligate nasal breathers and some infants with dacryoceles will present with respiratory distress secondary to a cystic bulging of the mucosa of the distal nasolacrimal duct into the nasal cavity. This may produce stridor or bilateral nasal airway obstruction. A computed tomography (CT) or magnetic resonance imaging (MRI) to demonstrate an intranasal cyst may be indicated in some cases.

Pathology

In a typical nasolacrimal duct obstruction, there is a distal obstruction or membrane at the valve of Hasner near the inferior meatus in the nasal cavity. In dacryoceles, there is a similar congenital distal membranous blockage of the nasolacrimal duct at the inferior meatus causing lacrimal sac distension, but also an obstruction of the entrance to the sac via the common canaliculus at the valve of Rosenmuller. Both antegrade and retrograde discharge of accumulated secretions is prevented, and a firm, distended lacrimal sac that feels hard is the result.

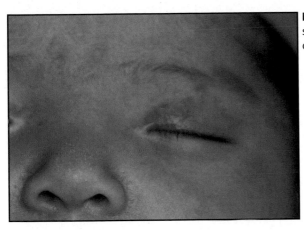

Figure 43-3. Same patient as in Figure 43-1 showing resolution of nasal mass following digital massage decompression.

Treatment

As mentioned previously, the management of dacryoceles involves an attempt to decompress the cyst with firm digital pressure. Using your index finger directed toward the nasal bone at the medial canthus, firmly press on the cyst and massage it. You may see clear or mucoid viscous fluid escape between the eyelids as the cyst decompresses. Continue to massage until the cyst reduces. This maneuver may be curative in over 50% of patients (Figure 43-3). The cyst may reform if the obstructions remain. If there is a visible discharge of mucus from the nose during massage, most likely the distal obstruction has been overcome and the dacryocele will be unlikely to reform. Nurses or caregivers should be instructed to perform digital massage regularly and briefly to prevent reformation of the cyst. This practice should be continued for a few days following decompression.

Some babies with congenital dacryoceles will require probing and irrigation of the nasolacrimal system for treatment if digital massage fails. Experienced pediatric ophthalmologists may choose to proceed with the probing at the bedside or in the clinic. Others may prefer to perform the procedure under general anesthesia and may elect to use nasal endoscopy to visualize an intranasal cyst that may be present. The probe may decompress the cyst in the nasal cavity, but some will require marsupialization of the mucocele under endoscopic guidance for definitive treatment.

The differential diagnosis of a mass in the typical location of a congenital dacryocele is limited. A capilliary hemangioma in this location is not present at birth but appears around 2 weeks of age and has a rubbery consistency upon palpation. Nasal dermoid or epidermoid cysts are not generally present in the perinatal period. A congenital encephalocele in this location would not be firm and might be reducible.

Suggested Readings

Dagi LR, Bhargava A, Melvin P. Associated sign, demographic characteristics, and management of dacryocystocele in 64 infants. *J AAPOS*. 2012;16:255-260.

Hain M, Bawnik Y, Warman M, et al. Neonatal dacryocele with endonasal cyst: revisiting the management. *Am J Otolaryngol*. 2011;32(2):152-155.

Wagner RS. Dacryocele. In: Maguire JI, Murchison AP, Jaeger EA, eds. *Wills Eye Institute 5-Minute Ophthalmology Consult*. Philadelphia, PA: Lippincott Williams & Wilkins;2012:236-237.

Wong RK, VanderVeen DK. Presentation and management of congenital dacryocystocele. *Pediatrics*. 2008;122:e1108-e1112.

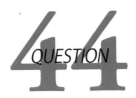

DO CHILDREN WITH EPIBLEPHARON AND TEARING REQUIRE EYELID SURGERY TO ALLEVIATE THEIR PROBLEM?

Renelle Pointdujour Lim, MD and Roman Shinder, MD

An epiblepharon is a congenital horizontal fold of skin near the margin of the lower eyelid caused by the abnormal insertion of muscle fibers, which causes the eyelashes to assume a vertical position (Figure 44-1). The condition is usually bilateral, and most prevalent in Asian children. The anatomical feature in epiblepharon is the absence of adhesion between lower lid structures, allowing the lid skin and underlying orbicularis muscle to roll upward. Like the upper lid, the main structural difference of the lower eyelid in Asians compared with Caucasians is the absence of a lower eyelid crease. This is why epiblepharon is more common in Asian children.

There are several possible etiologic factors contributing to the pathogenesis of epiblepharon, including failure of lower eyelid retractor muscles gaining access to the overlying skin; failure of proper septal connections in the subcutaneous plane; and weak attachment of the orbicularis oculi muscle and lid skin to the deep layers of the lid, thus raising a skin fold near the eyelid margin and directing the lower lid lashes in an abnormal vertical direction.

Most times, epiblepharon are asymptomatic even when the lashes touch the cornea, and such patients may be observed. Many cases resolve over time with the normal growth of facial features (Figure 44-2). Few patients demonstrate constant clinical symptoms, whereas others are symptomatic only in downgaze when the lashes rub the eye. The aberrant eyelashes may rub against the cornea, producing a foreign body sensation, photophobia, tearing, discharge, conjunctival injection, blinking, pain, or eye rubbing. If the condition persists, corneal abrasion, keratitis, and permanent, visually significant corneal scarring may occur. Although the majority of patients can be managed conservatively, treatment should not be delayed in symptomatic cases. Even mild symptoms such as tearing should not be ignored and surgical correction should be offered to all symptomatic patients despite conservative lubrication of the eye with ointment. In the preoperative

Wagner R. *Curbside Consultation in Pediatric Ophthalmology: 49 Clinical Questions* (pp 211-214)
© 2014 SLACK Incorporated

Figure 44-1. (A-C) Examples of epiblepharon. Note the vertical orientation of the lower lid lashes.

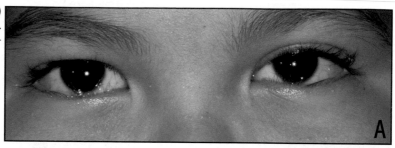

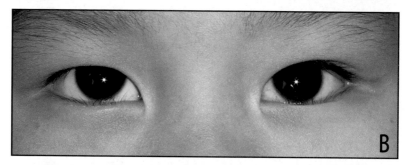

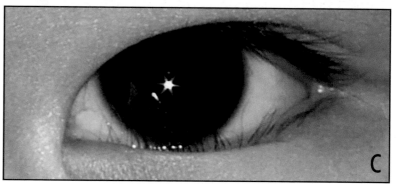

period, parents should be instructed to use ophthalmic ointment to the symptomatic eye to act as a corneal barrier to improve symptomatology and decrease the risk of corneal damage.

A few other conditions may mimic epiblepharon, so it is important to accurately distinguish them. The most common considerations to rule out when evaluating a child with suspected epiblepharon are distichiasis and trichiasis. Distichiasis occurs when an abnormal additional row of lashes arises from the posterior lid margin. The eyelashes emerge from an abnormal posterior position of the lid margin, whereas in epiblepharon the lashes originate from the normal anterior lid margin location. Potential causes of distichiasis include congenital, traumatic, or iatrogenic from prior lid surgery. In congenital distichiasis, the lashes are directed posteriorly toward the ocular surface and may not become symptomatic until about 5 years of age, whereas epiblepharon generally improves with time.

Unlike epiblepharon, which is a congenital condition, trichiasis is an acquired condition in which lashes arise from their normal anterior lid margin position and are misdirected toward the ocular surface. This often results from inflammation and scarring of the eyelash follicles, as seen in conditions such as blepharitis and ocular rosacea.

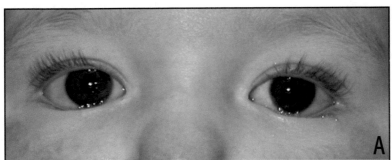

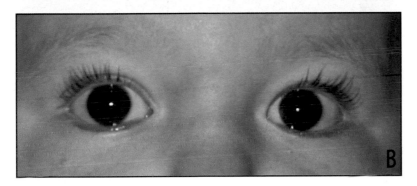

Figure 44-2. (A) Epiblepharon at initial presentation. (B) Improvement after 4 months of observation.

Treatment

The object of surgical treatment for epiblepharon is to eliminate the abnormal lower lid skin fold and thereby orient the lashes in a more normal anatomic direction away from the eye. There are several techniques used; however, we will describe our preferred procedure. Excision of the skin fold and an underlying strip of orbicularis muscle has traditionally been the most commonly performed procedure for epiblepharon. By excising these tissues and suturing the resultant defect, the lower eyelid margin rotates away from the globe and thus orients the lashes away from the eye. The incision is a subciliary approach just below the lower lid margin, which produces a cosmetically favorable scar and avoids creating a lower eyelid crease in an Asian child who would not typically have such a crease (Figure 44-3). This procedure is simple and has a high success rate. However, care must be taken not to remove too much tissue because lower eyelid retraction or ectropion may result.

Conclusion

If a child with epiblepharon is seen on routine examination, the child should be referred to an ophthalmologist, preferably a pediatric ophthalmologist or oculoplastic surgeon, for prompt evaluation. Most children are asymptomatic and can be observed. Symptomatic patients should receive ophthalmic ointment to protect the cornea, and serial ophthalmic examinations are warranted to document improved symptoms and lack of corneal damage. If symptoms persist or corneal pathology is noted despite lubrication, surgical intervention is indicated.

Figure 44-3. (A) Epiblepharon at initial presentation. (B) One week after surgical correction.

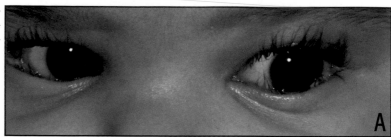

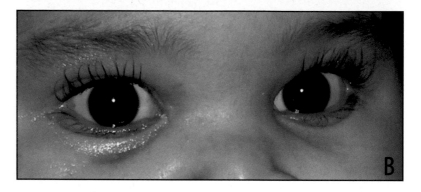

Suggested Readings

Jung J, Kim HK, Choi HY. Epiblepharon correction combined with skin redraping epicanthoplasty in children. *Craniofac Surg.* 2011;22(3):1024-1026.

Naik MN, Ali MJ, Das S, et al. Nonsurgical management of epiblepharon using hyaluronic acid gel. *Ophthal Plast Reconstr Surg.* 2010;26(3):215-217.

Woo KI, Yi K, Kim YD. Surgical correction for lower lid epiblepharon in Asians. *Br J Ophthalmol.* 2000;84:1407-1410.

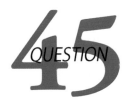

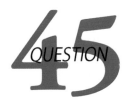QUESTION

45

WHAT ARE THE SIGNS AND SYMPTOMS OF CONGENITAL GLAUCOMA?

Catherine A. Origlieri, MD and Albert S. Khouri, MD

Primary congenital glaucoma is a rare but visually devastating ophthalmic condition that you may encounter during your career. In most instances, congenital glaucoma carries a poor prognosis, so the best management begins with prompt recognition and diagnosis. The goal of this chapter is to help you recognize the presenting signs and symptoms of this condition.

How Does Glaucoma Inflict Damage on the Visual System?

It is believed that elevated intraocular pressure (IOP) leads to optic nerve damage and therefore progressive loss of vision. In the pediatric population, the risk of visual loss from glaucoma is heightened by the immaturity of the visual system; thus children with congenital glaucoma may lose vision not only from the physiologic changes associated with glaucoma itself, but also from amblyopia. Congenital glaucoma occurs in 1:10,000 to 30,000 live births and may exist sporadically or from a genetic predisposition. Some forms of congenital glaucoma are associated with systemic syndromes, which are discussed next.

When evaluating a patient with glaucoma, you should be familiar with the terminology used to describe the various forms of glaucoma that you might encounter in the pediatric population (Table 45-1). Based on the age at presentation, the terms *newborn* or *birth-onset congenital glaucoma* (less than 1 month of age), *infantile-onset primary congenital glaucoma* (between 1 month and 2 years), and *late-onset* or *late-recognized primary infantile glaucoma* (older than 2 years) are used. The majority of patients present between a few months and 2 years of age. These distinctions

Wagner R. *Curbside Consultation in Pediatric Ophthalmology: 49 Clinical Questions* (pp 215-220)
© 2014 SLACK Incorporated

Table 45-1
Classification of Pediatric Glaucoma

Primary Glaucoma	Secondary Glaucoma
Newborn/birth-onset	Uveitis
Infantile-onset	Ocular neoplasm: retinoblastoma
Late-onset/late-recognized	Systemic/ophthalmic steroids
Juvenile open-angle	Trauma
	Lens dislocation
	Neovascularization
	Intraocular infection
	Complications from congenital cataract extraction

are mostly arbitrary and observational and do not have a significant bearing on management. It is important, however, to keep in mind that all of the above are forms of primary congenital glaucoma and should not be confused with *juvenile open-angle glaucoma,* an autosomal-dominant condition found in older children and young adults that is often managed similarly to adult glaucomas. Likewise, is it important to distinguish primary glaucomas from secondary glaucomas that occur as a result of other factors, such as uveitis, steroid use, or trauma.

Why Does High Intraocular Pressure Develop?

Now that you have a more accurate understanding of how to categorize congenital glaucoma, we can discuss the pathophysiology, signs, and symptoms of this condition. It is believed that eyes with primary congenital glaucoma have undergone erroneous or incomplete development of the anterior eye structures during fetal life. In a normal eye, the trabecular meshwork, located in the angle formed by the junction of the iris and cornea, is the main outlet for intraocular fluid. Neural crest cells are responsible for the formation of this trabecular meshwork. Thus, improper development and function of this structure lead to accumulation of aqueous humor within the eye and increased IOP. If this elevation in pressure is sustained, the outcome is direct and irreversible damage to the optic nerve. Interestingly, in addition to forming the trabecular meshwork, neural crest cells are also responsible for the development of the corneal endothelium, corneal keratocytes, and iris stroma. In many forms of congenital glaucoma, these structures are also abnormal.

Primary congenital glaucoma is bilateral in most cases, although the onset and severity may be asymmetric. In one-fourth of patients, signs are present at birth. Some of the more obvious signs and symptoms involve the cornea. Therefore, you should always examine the front of an infant's eye to evaluate for these findings. One of the most striking signs of congenital glaucoma is *corneal edema,* which you may recognize as a hazy, grayish, or opaque appearance to the normally clear cornea (Figure 45-1). Corneal edema occurs because corneal endothelial cells in eyes with high IOP cannot provide a proper barrier against the influx of intraocular fluid into the corneal stroma. Under normal IOP, the endothelial cells keep the cornea dehydrated and clear. Furthermore, the basement membrane of corneal endothelial cells can rupture when exposed to persistently elevated

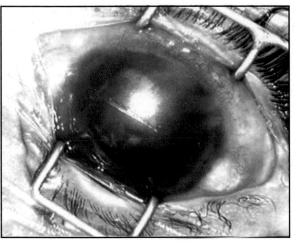

Figure 45-1. Corneal edema in congenital glaucoma.

IOP, allowing even more fluid to infiltrate the cornea. These breaks in Descemet's membrane, called *Haab's striae*, appear as horizontal or concentric fine lines or scars within the cornea (only appreciated with biomicroscopy). They are different from the more vertical or oblique tears in Descemet's membrane commonly seen after birth trauma.

What Are the Signs and Symptoms?

Traditionally, the triad associated with congenital glaucoma includes epiphora (tearing), photophobia, and blepharospasm. Corneal edema is the main reason for epiphora and photophobia frequently observed in infants with congenital glaucoma. The presence of corneal edema is irritating and painful to the patient; the conjunctiva in these eyes may also appear injected. The hazy edematous cornea creates a light-scattering effect, which exacerbates the above symptoms. Tearing in the newborn is quite common and usually indicates a more benign and much more common condition such as nasolacrimal duct obstruction or *dacrocystocele*. It is important, however, for you to recognize that tearing may also be a sign of congenital glaucoma, particularly in the setting of corneal edema, which is not seen in babies with nasolacrimal duct abnormalities.

Megalocornea, or enlarged corneal diameter, is another sign of congenital glaucoma (Figure 45-2). A normal newborn horizontal corneal diameter measures 9.5 to 10.5 mm and reaches normal adult size of 12.0 mm by 2 to 3 years of age. Collagen in the newborn eye, specifically in the cornea and sclera, is more distensible than in the adult eye. For this reason, elevated IOP in an infant with glaucoma can literally alter the size and shape of the eye. In fact, these children not only have abnormally enlarged corneas but may also have larger-than-normal eyes. The term *buphthalmos*, meaning "ox eye," refers to the enlarged globe typical of infants with congenital glaucoma. These eyes are prone to axial myopia because the longer shape of the eye induces nearsightedness. Megalocornea or buphthalmos may be difficult to recognize in a patient with bilateral congenital glaucoma because both eyes may be symmetrically enlarged.

In patients with clear corneas, you should attempt to examine the optic nerve with a direct ophthalmoscope. Patients with congenital glaucoma frequently have *optic nerve cupping* (Figure 45-3). A normal cup-to-disc ratio in an infant is typically 0.3 or less. A ratio larger than 0.3 should raise suspicion for optic nerve pathology. However, keep in mind that the optic nerve can normally have a cup-to-disc ratio greater than 0.3 and that there are other nonglaucomatous conditions (eg, optic nerve coloboma or optic nerve hypoplasia) that can also alter the appearance of the optic disc.

Figure 45-2. Asymmetric megalocornea in a patient with congenital glaucoma.

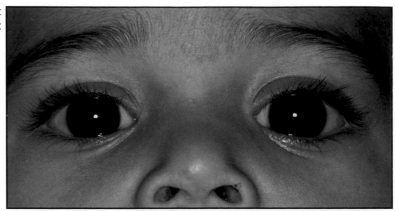

Figure 45-3. Optic nerve cupping.

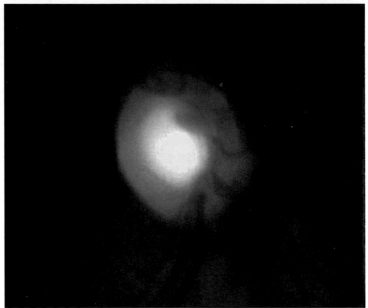

Unlike cases of adult glaucoma, infants with congenital glaucoma may demonstrate some degree of reversal in optic disc cupping once IOP is controlled. However, damage to the optic nerve is, for the most part irreversible, leading to permanent loss of vision and blindness in untreated eyes.

Any of the previous signs and symptoms can occur in the setting of congenital glaucoma. In many such cases, congenital glaucoma occurs as an isolated finding in an otherwise healthy patient; in other instances, congenital glaucoma may be part of an ocular or systemic condition or syndrome (Table 45-2). *Sturge-Weber syndrome,* or encephalotrigeminal angiomatosis, carries an approximately 30% risk of glaucoma, with two-thirds of such patients exhibiting signs of glaucoma by age 2 years. Increased IOP in patients with Sturge-Weber syndrome may occur from either abnormal angle anatomy or increased episcleral venous pressure due to abnormal vasculature. Involvement of the upper eyelid by a vascular nevus is directly correlated with the incidence of glaucoma in these patients. In fact, almost 50% of children with a port-wine stain involving the first or second division of the trigeminal nerve develop ipsilateral glaucoma.

Another systemic syndrome associated with pediatric glaucoma is the autosomal-dominant condition *neurofibromatosis type 1* (NF1), or *von Recklinghausen's disease.* Patients with NF1 are

Table 45-2

Congenital Glaucoma Associated With Ocular and Systemic Abnormalities

Congenital Ocular Anomalies	*Systemic Syndromes*
Aniridia	Autosomal-dominant:
Microcornea	Neurofibromatosis type I
Sclerocornea	Sticklers' syndrome
Microcoria	Oculodentodigital dysplasia
Microphthalmos	Osteogenesis imperfecta
Iridotrabecular dysgenesis	Axenfeld-Rieger syndrome
Peters' anomaly	Marfan syndrome
Persistent hyperplastic primary vitreous	Open-angle glaucoma associated with microcornea and absent frontal sinuses
Posterior polymorphous dystrophy	Kneist dysplasia
Congenital ocular melanosis (nevus of Ota)	Michels syndrome
	Autosomal-recessive:
	Zellweger (hepatocerebrorenal) syndrome
	Mucopolysaccharidosis (except MPS II)
	Cystinosis
	Warburg's syndrome
	X-linked recessive:
	Lowe (oculocerebrorenal) syndrome
	Hunter's syndrome (MPS II)
	Sporadic:
	Sturge-Weber syndrome
	Rubenstein-Taybi syndrome
	Chromosomal trisomies (eg, 13 and 18)
	Chromosomal deletions (eg, Turner syndrome)
	Cutis marmorata telangiectasia congenita
	Prader-Willi syndrome
	Krause's syndrome

thought to develop glaucoma due to abnormal angle anatomy. The presence of a plexiform neuro-fibroma of the upper eyelid is associated with ipsilateral glaucoma in approximately 50% of cases. Other ocular findings in patients with NF1 include iris Lisch nodules and optic nerve gliomas.

All children with congenital glaucoma, whether occurring in isolation or in conjunction with a systemic syndrome, should be diagnosed as early as possible so that the appropriate measures can be taken to reduce the risk of visual loss. Early recognition of the signs and symptoms are key to early intervention. Siblings of affected children should be screened for ocular and systemic conditions associated with congenital glaucoma. As physicians, it is also important that we remain cognizant of the heavy burden this condition and its prolonged follow-up bears on patients, their parents, and caregivers. As a caregiver to pediatric patients, you can play a pivotal role in the detection and collaborative care of this potentially blinding condition.

Suggested Readings

Hylton C, Beck A. Congenital glaucoma and other childhood glaucomas. In: Shaarawy TM, Sherwood MB, Hitchings RA, Crowston JG, eds. *Glaucoma Volume 1: Medical Diagnosis & Therapy.* China: Elsevier Limited; 2009:369-381.

Mattox C, Walton DS. Hereditary primary childhood glaucomas. *Int Ophthalmol Clin.* 1993;33:121-134.

Olitsky SE. Primary infantile glaucoma. *Int Ophthalmol Clin.* 2010;50(4):57-66.

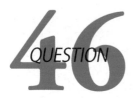

QUESTION

HOW OFTEN SHOULD CHILDREN WITH JUVENILE IDIOPATHIC ARTHRITIS BE SEEN BY THE OPHTHALMOLOGIST?

David S. Chu, MD

Juvenile idiopathic arthritis (JIA) is an autoimmune disease that can affect children of any age. It is also known as *juvenile rheumatoid arthritis, juvenile chronic arthritis,* or *Still's disease.* As the name implies, arthritis is the most frequent presenting symptom and clinical feature in patients afflicted with JIA. The eye is the most common extra-articular site of manifestation. In the eyes, JIA patients most commonly present with anterior uveitis. Identifying signs of ocular involvement can be more challenging in pediatric patients compared with adults because the involved eyes generally do not appear red, children usually don't complain of symptoms, and they are more difficult to examine.

The course and severity of uveitis can vary greatly and may not follow any particular pattern. Uveitis is one of the most common causes of irreversible blindness in children. Many options exist for effective treatment of uveitis in children with JIA; however, if not recognized promptly or treated properly, loss of sight is a common scenario. A review of the literature, as well as my own clinical experience, has shown that when children present to uveitis specialists with impaired vision from the complication of uveitis, they generally do not regain the lost sight.

As mentioned previously, the most common ocular manifestation of JIA is uveitis more specifically *nongranulomatous anterior uveitis.* Through slit-lamp examination, the physician can identify circulating inflammatory cells in the anterior chamber of the eye. In addition to anterior uveitis, other forms of ocular inflammation may also be seen, including conjunctivitis, scleritis, posterior uveitis, and papillitis. Other ophthalmic findings as the consequence of uveitis include band keratopathy, cataract, glaucoma, iris synechiae, macular edema, or retinal detachment. Typically, the inflamed eye does not exhibit any external sign of inflammation (redness or local edema) to the naked eye (Figure 46-1). Moreover, patients may be asymptomatic. Even when the inflammation is severe enough to be symptomatic or there are sight-threatening complications of ocular

Wagner R. *Curbside Consultation in Pediatric Ophthalmology: 49 Clinical Questions* (pp 221-223)
© 2014 SLACK Incorporated

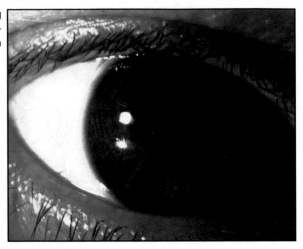

Figure 46-1. White, uninflamed-appearing eye with anterior uveitis and posterior synechiae and uveitic cataract, typically seen in patients with JIA.

inflammation such as cataract, glaucoma, or retinal detachment or edema, children may not report any symptoms to caregivers or offer any complaint to physicians if they are too young to communicate. Even if they are capable of communicating, patients may ignore the symptoms and find ways to cope with their limitations. Examination of younger children poses a special challenge, because cooperation may be absent, and examination may require anesthesia.

Risk factors for uveitis in JIA include pauciarticular subtype, positive serum antinuclear antibody (ANA), female sex, and early onset (younger than 6 years old), whereas polyarticular subtype and positive rheumatoid factor (RF) appear negatively correlated. JIA affects children from all ethnic backgrounds; however, the published literature on the epidemiology are mostly from the United States and northern Europe. Data vary greatly with respect to the occurrence of uveitis in JIA, ranging from 5% to 24%.

Various recommendations on frequency of monitoring exist. A group from Finland recommended that all JIA patients be evaluated by an ophthalmologist experienced with uveitis at the time of diagnosis, after which high-risk patients should be evaluated every 3 months for 2 years and then every 6 months for at least 7 years. Other subgroups are to be evaluated annually. This is a reasonable recommendation, and in my practice I follow similar guidelines. Children without risk factors but who are treated with systemic steroids are followed more frequently than every 6 months because of potential ocular complications, namely cataracts, which may result in amblyopia in children younger than 8 years old.

Conclusion

JIA is the systemic condition most commonly associated with childhood uveitis. Uveitis remains one of the most frequent causes of irreversible blindness. There are many effective and safe treatment options. Children with JIA should receive timely screening by an ophthalmologist experienced in caring for these patients, and if any ocular inflammation is seen, they are to be treated swiftly to ensure the best visual outcome.

Suggested Readings

Kanski JJ. Juvenile arthritis and uveitis. *Surv Ophthalmol.* 1990;34(4):253-267.

Kesen MR, Setlur V, Goldstein DA. Juvenile idiopathic arthritis-related uveitis. *Int Ophthalmol Clin.* 2008;48(3):21-38.

Kotaniemi K, Savolainen A, Karma A, Aho K. Recent advances in uveitis of juvenile idiopathic arthritis. *Surv Ophthalmol.* 2003;48(5):489-502.

Kump LI, Cervantes-Castañeda RA, Androudi SN, Foster CS. Analysis of pediatric uveitis cases at a tertiary referral center. *Ophthalmology.* 2005;112(7):1287-1292.

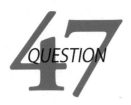

Does Congenital Ptosis Cause Amblyopia in Many Cases?

William R. Katowitz, MD

Congenital ptosis can cause amblyopia, especially in cases where the pupil covers the central visual axis (deprivation amblyopia). The reported incidence of amblyopia in individuals with ptosis ranges from 17% to 71%.[1,2] Furthermore, it has been shown that children with congenital ptosis have a risk of strabismic and anisometropic amblyopia.[3] Thus, it is critical to thoroughly work-up all children with ptosis for all risk factors of amblyopia. This involves a dilated eye examination in addition to the external examination of the face and eyelid function.

It is easy to overlook the congenital third nerve palsy in a patient if you focus solely on the eyelids and proceed with ptosis surgery alone. This patient, who would be at risk for deprivation amblyopia, would also require patching or cycloplegic therapy and possible strabismus surgery.

Amblyopia Screening

It is critical to document the severity of ptosis. I often ask parents to bring photos of their child, especially in cases where there is a report of variability to the ptosis. In some instances such as birth trauma or even myasthenia gravis of infancy, the ptosis can improve with time. Examining the child with congenital ptosis can be extremely challenging. All too often a child is completely asleep during the examination. One of the easiest tricks to examine infants who have their eyes closed is to dim the examination room light. This will often elicit an eye-popping reflex, where an infant will open his or her eyes in response to a darkened room light. I often set my flash to ready when photographing a patient and, when dimming the lights, take a picture to document the patient's eyelid height. In these instances, assessing levator function can be too difficult and should be repeated in a follow-up examination.

Wagner R. *Curbside Consultation in Pediatric
Ophthalmology: 49 Clinical Questions* (pp 225-227)
© 2014 SLACK Incorporated

Figure 47-1. Schematic comparing ptosis (in mm) to MRD1. (Adapted from Katowitz JA, ed. *Pediatric Oculoplastic Surgery.* New York, NY: Springer-Verlag; 2002:260. Used with kind permission of Springer Science+Business Media.)

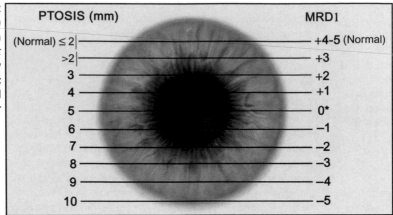

PTOSIS (mm)	MRD1
(Normal) ≤2	+4-5 (Normal)
>2	+3
3	+2
4	+1
5	0*
6	−1
7	−2
8	−3
9	−4
10	−5

Assessing an infant's vision is also challenging. Some physicians rely on *visual evoked potential* (VEP) electrophysiology testing to screen for amblyopia.[4] However, this is time intensive and requires a dedicated lab for testing. At the Children's Hospital of Philadelphia, we rely on Teller visual acuity cards, but this test is not accurate until a child is at least 3 months of age.[5] Any signs of a visual preference either noted on cover testing or a documented difference in visual acuity in the setting of ptosis should alert an evaluator that a patient with ptosis may suffer from amblyopia. In addition, an accurate refraction to screen for anisometropia and for large refractive errors is necessary and can be accomplished in an office without the need for sedation.

Measuring Ptosis

It is important to have a system to describe the severity of ptosis. Some physicians report, "This patient has 3 mm of ptosis." The problem with this phrase is that it is open ended. Is this referring to the difference between the eyelids or the amount of droop relative to the limbus? A better system to measure the amount of ptosis is that of the distance (in mm) from the eyelid margin to the center of the pupil (or central light reflex). Figure 47-1 depicts the different ways to quantify eyelid ptosis. The *margin reflex distance* (MRD) can then be measured for each eyelid (MRD[1] for upper and MRD[2] for lower).

Margin Reflex Distance and Amblyopia

A patient born with an eyelid at or below the central visual axis is at risk for central vision loss due to the lack of visual stimulus *(deprivation amblyopia).* The timing and choice for surgical repair is addressed in Question 48. Some patients with severe ptosis (MRD of 0 or less) do not have amblyopia, and this is most likely due to the fact that they are able to recruit the frontalis muscle to lift the eyelid, as well as to see under their lid with a chin up position.

Congenital ptosis can cause amblyopia, and this should be considered in severe cases. It is reasonable to proceed with ptosis surgery in any child who is at risk for amblyopia due to ptosis, even when it is too early to assess the vision quantitatively.

References

1. Fiergang DL, Wright KW, Foster JA. Unilateral or asymmetric congenital ptosis, head posturing, and amblyopia. *J Pediatr Ophthalmol Strabismus.* 1999;36:74-77.
2. Harrad RA, Graham CM, Collin JR. Amblyopia and strabismus in congenital ptosis. *Eye (Lond).* 1988;2:625-627.
3. Srinagesh V, Simon, JW, Meyer DR, Zobal-Ratner J. The association of refractive error, strabismus, and amblyopia with congenital ptosis. *J AAPOS.* 2011;15:541-544.
4. McCulloch DL, Wright KW. Unilateral congenital ptosis: compensatory head posturing and amblyopia. *Ophthal Plast Reconstr Surg.* 1993;9(3):196-200.
5. Drover JR, Wyatt LM, Stager DR, Birch EE. The teller acuity cards are effective in detecting amblyopia. *Optom Vis Sci.* 2009;86(6):755-759.

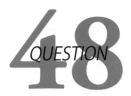

WHICH CHILDREN WITH CONGENITAL PTOSIS USUALLY REQUIRE SURGERY?

William R. Katowitz, MD

When approaching a child with congenital ptosis, it is critical to ask the correct questions. What is the cause of the ptosis? What is the severity of the ptosis? Is the vision impaired, and does it threaten proper visual development? The overall well-being of the child is paramount. Thus, focusing solely on a droopy eyelid without thoroughly exploring the cause of this droop could have grave consequences. You would not want to miss, for example, the patient with mild ptosis, who also has anisometropia and a neuroblastoma metastatic to the neck inducing Horner syndrome.

Diagnosis

Identifying the etiology of ptosis is critical. The most common isolated congenital ptosis should be a diagnosis of exclusion after you have carefully ruled out other causes. A thorough history and examination can direct you toward the most likely diagnosis. This begins with a family history as well as a birth history. Is there ptosis in your family? Does anyone in your family have blepharophimosis syndrome or orbital fibrosis? How was your child delivered? Were forceps used? Was your child's eyelid (or eyelids) droopy at birth? Does your child's eyelid jump when feeding? All of these are helpful questions.

A special consideration must be directed toward the acquired mechanical ptosis seen in infancy due to capillary hemangioma. These lesions, when in the orbit or eyebrow, can infiltrate the eyelid, inducing a ptotic eyelid that can block the central visual axis. Fortunately, there are nonsurgical treatments (eg, oral beta blocker therapy) that can produce an exquisite response.[1] Figure 48-1A shows a 4-month-old boy with a right orbital hemangioma and ptosis. Figure 48-1B is the same child only 3 months after oral beta blocker therapy. In the past, this is a patient who may have

Wagner R. *Curbside Consultation in Pediatric
Ophthalmology: 49 Clinical Questions* (pp 229-232)
© 2014 SLACK Incorporated

Figure 48-1. (A) A 4-month-old boy with a right orbital hemangioma and ptosis. (B) Three months after oral beta-blocker therapy.

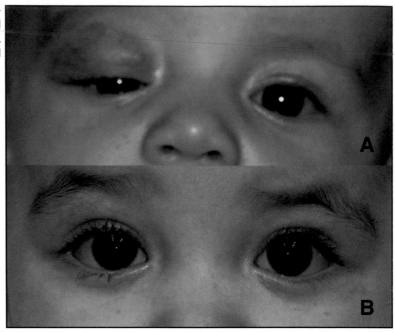

required surgical intervention if steroid therapy failed. Please keep in mind that a patient with a large, superficial segmental hemangioma should be screened for posterior fossa malformations, hemangiomas, arterial anomalies, cardiac defects, eye abnormalities, sternal cleft, and supraumbilical raphe (PHACES) syndrome before being started on oral beta blocker therapy due to the risk of stroke.

Several examination findings factor into the description of the severity of ptosis. The measurement of eyelid height in mm from the center of the cornea to the upper eyelid marginal reflex distance (MRD[1]) was discussed in Question 47. Levator function should be measured without brow use. I typically use a short, child-friendly video on my smartphone as a fixation device when examining a child in up gaze and down gaze. When you see the cornea buried under a ptotic eyelid in up gaze, this should alert you that the levator function is likely poor. Excessive chin up position should also be noted because this should factor into the description of ptosis severity. Keep in mind that the drive to maintain binocular vision is strong, and if there is a chin up face position that accomplishes this, even infants will develop ocular torticollis. Ocular motility and alignment and Bell's phenomenon are important to note. In the setting of double elevator palsy or any up gaze deficit, it is important to be aware of the risk of exposure keratopathy after ptosis surgery. A careful refraction should be obtained. The weight of a ptotic eyelid can deform the globe, inducing with-the-rule astigmatism.[2] Finally, the presence of strabismus is an opportunity to visit the concept of combined eye muscle and ptosis surgery. Sometimes a delay in ptosis surgery can be made until you decide to proceed with strabismus repair as a combined procedure after failed nonsurgical interventions for strabismus (such as glasses).

Management

Classically, one may think of an MRD[1] that encroaches upon or covers the central visual axis as having the greatest potential to threaten visual development. If we are to assume the average

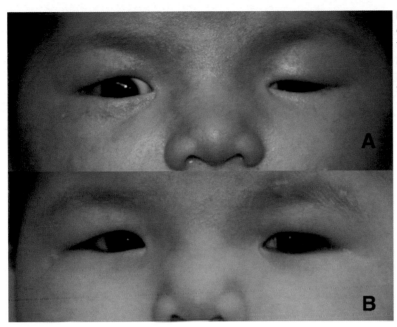

Figure 48-2. (A) A 6-week-old girl with congenital third nerve palsy and a left MRD[1] of 0. (B) Two months postoperative from silicone frontalis sling surgery.

pupil size in photopic (well-lit) conditions is 3 to 4 mm, this would mean an MRD[1] of 1.5 mm or less is severely amblyogenic.[3] A chin up face position may be protective against the development of deprivation amblyopia. Figure 48-2A shows a 6-week-old girl with congenital third nerve palsy and a left MRD[1] of 0. Figure 48-2B is the same child 2 months postoperative from silicone frontalis sling surgery.

More critical than MRD[1] alone, however, is the symmetry between the eyelids. This is perhaps what we notice the most in each other's eyelids. It is important not to just treat a number but rather the person. I have found that patients, parents, and pediatricians are alarmed when they note eyelid asymmetry and sometimes request ptosis surgery even when the eyelid height is not amblyogenic. Currently, insurance companies consider ptosis that is not vision threatening as purely cosmetic. What is not appreciated, however, is the potential for a child to experience body dysmorphism due to his or her eyelid asymmetry. Other children certainly can bring this to their attention. "What's wrong with your eye?" is a common question pediatric patients with ptosis are asked by their peers. This leads to the controversy of whether we should consider ptosis surgery in a pediatric patient as both vision saving and preserving appearance. Certainly the severe ptosis seen in Figure 48-2 warrants prompt surgical repair, but what about the patient with mild ptosis due to Horner syndrome? I never thrust surgery upon patients and families. First, ptosis surgery can be a large commitment for caregivers. For example, the patient in Figure 48-2 required frequent eye lubrication to prevent corneal exposure. Second, not all patients or families perceive ptosis the same way. Some parents feel strongly that if the ptosis is not vision threatening, it should not be performed, whereas others see a 1-mm asymmetry as disfiguring.

In the setting of ptosis, any evidence of amblyopia should be treated, such as a gaze preference, strabismus, or documented poor vision. This can include glasses, patching, or atropine. Moderate to mild ptosis with amblyopia (MRD[1] of 1.5 mm or greater) can be managed without surgical intervention; however, you can argue that repairing the ptosis in this setting would be the most effective amblyopia therapy.

The timing of surgical repair is also controversial. Although most ophthalmologists agree that severe ptosis requires early intervention, many patients with moderate to mild ptosis are followed until at least the age of 4 years. In this approach, surgery is deferred until better measurements and a more reliable visual acuity can be obtained.[4] At the Children's Hospital of Philadelphia, we prefer to delay elective ptosis repairs until after the age of 6 months due to the risks of general anesthesia but intervene sometime after this, typically around the age of 1 year. We feel earlier intervention is less emotionally traumatic for the unaware infant and less challenging to the parents who have to care for them postoperatively.[5]

Not all children with congenital ptosis will require surgical intervention, but in my experience, most children will eventually want it. Should this factor into our decision making when consulting parents? I think it should. That being said, surgery can always be deferred when good vision is documented in both eyes and patients (and parents) are otherwise happy with their appearance. Ptosis surgery is, after all, meant to treat the patient and not the surgeon.

References

1. Léauté-Labrèze C, Dumas de la Roque E, Hubiche T, Boralevi F, Thambo JB, Taïeb A. Propranolol for severe hemangiomas of infancy. *N Engl J Med*. 2008;12;358(24):2649-2651.
2. Harrad RA, Graham CM, Collin JRO. Amblyopia and strabismus in congenital ptosis. In: *Ptosis*. 4th ed. Birmingham, AL: Aesculapius; 1990:113-167.
3. Kobashi H, Kamiya K, Ishikawa H, Goseki T, Shimizu K. Daytime variations in pupil size under photopic conditions. *Optom Vis Sci*. 2012;89(2):197-202.
4. Iliff CE. Problems in ptosis surgery. In: Rycroft PV, ed. *Corneo-plastic Surgery*. Oxford, UK: Pergamon; 1969:15-29.
5. Heher KL, Katowitz JA. Pediatric ptosis. In: Katowitz JA, ed. *Pediatric Oculoplastic Surgery*. New York, NY: Springer-Verlag; 2002:253-288.

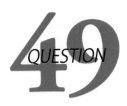

WHAT IS BLEPHAROPHIMOSIS SYNDROME, AND HOW IS IT MANAGED?

Paul D. Langer, MD, FACS

Blepharophimosis syndrome (or, more formally, *blepharophimosis-ptosis-epicanthus inversus syndrome* [BPES]) is a congenital, autosomal-dominantly inherited condition characterized by the presence of 4 complex eyelid anomalies:

1. *Epicanthus inversus* (an abnormal fold of skin extending medially and superiorly from the lower eyelid to cover the medial commissure)

2. *Telecanthus* (an increased distance between the medial canthi in the presence of a normal intrapupillary distance)

3. *Severe blepharoptosis*

4. *Blepharophimosis* (a horizontal narrowing of the palpebral apertures)

In addition, children with this condition have excess subcutaneous tissue in the medial canthal area and a flat nasal bridge, the combination of which leads to a loss of the natural concavity of the medial canthi. Other clinical features commonly seen include ectropion of the lateral portion of the lower eyelids, low-set ears, and a short philtrum.

Two variations of BPES are recognized. Type I is associated with premature ovarian failure and infertility in women, whereas type II is not associated with ovarian disease. Genetic testing reveals an abnormality in the *FOXL2* gene (located on chromosome 3) in over 80% of cases of both types.[1]

Surgical management of the condition requires two distinct procedures: one to correct the medial canthal deformities and one to address the ptotic upper eyelids. A number of techniques have been described to reconstruct the medial canthus in BPES, all of which aim to eliminate the epicanthal fold and shorten the medial canthal tendon (which reduces the telecanthus and improves the phimosis). In all cases, a frontalis sling procedure is required to adequately raise the eyelids to an acceptable height because the function of the levator palpebrae superioris muscle is

Wagner R. *Curbside Consultation in Pediatric Ophthalmology: 49 Clinical Questions* (pp 233-235)
© 2014 SLACK Incorporated

Figure 49-1. (A) Preoperative photograph of a child with blepharophimosis. (B) Intraoperative photograph detailing inner canthal drawings for five-flap technique. *(continued)*

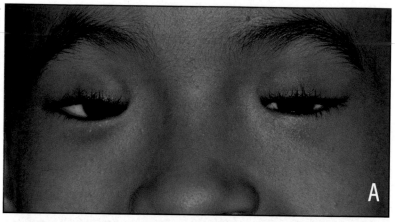

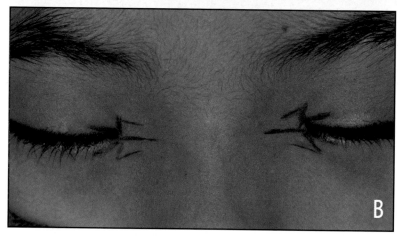

significantly reduced in this condition. Some surgeons prefer to perform both procedures simultaneously, whereas others perform them independently. Because a shortening of the medial canthal tendon pulls both the upper and lower eyelids medially under significant tension and a frontalis sling procedure exerts significant force on the upper eyelid superiorly, I separate the 2 surgeries to avoid pulling the upper eyelid in 2 directions simultaneously, allowing for more predictable surgical results.

The medial canthal procedure I prefer is the "five-flap" technique as described by Anderson and Nowinski.[2] This technique combines a Y-to-V-plasty with 2 Z-plasties on each side. In essence, a Y-to-V-plasty converts a Y incision over the medial commissure into a V at closure. In pulling the central point of the Y incision toward the apex to create a V, the technique pulls the medial commissure toward the nose, reducing telecanthus and widening the palpebral aperture. Two critical aspects of this maneuver are the resection of the excess subcutaneous tissue of the medial canthus and the plication of the medial canthal tendon medially and posteriorly, which together restore the natural concavity of the medial canthal area. The 2 Z-plasties serve to eliminate the epicanthal fold and allow for easier transposition of tissue (Figure 49-1).

Because the ptosis in BPES is bilateral and symmetric, the majority of children with this condition do not develop amblyopia. Therefore, in most cases, I will first perform the medial canthal "five-flap" surgery at the age of 2 or 3 years and then perform a frontalis sling procedure 1 or 2 years later. If amblyopia develops, I will accelerate this timetable to raise the eyelids earlier in coordination with the recommendations of a pediatric ophthalmologist.

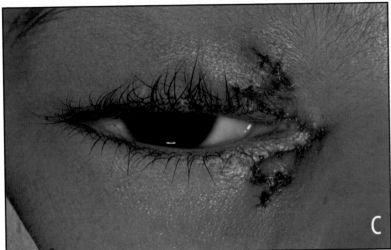

Figure 49-1. (continued) (C) Intraoperative photograph of right inner canthus following removal of excess medial canthal subcutaneous tissue, medial canthal tendon plication, and transposition of flaps. (D) Eight-month postoperative photograph.

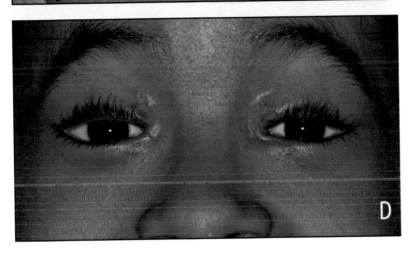

Parents of a child with blepharophimosis syndrome should receive genetic counseling if they are not already familiar with the disease or its inheritance pattern. De novo mutations are estimated to account for 50% or more of all cases, so many cases occur in families unfamiliar with the disease, despite the condition being transmitted in an autosomal-dominant fashion.[1] Girls affected with BPES should undergo endocrinologic and gynecologic monitoring later in life if they are suspected to have type I or if the type of BPES is unknown. Otherwise, children born with blepharophimosis syndrome would be expected to have normal intelligence and a natural lifespan. Subsequently, each offspring of a patient with BPES has a 50% chance of inheriting the condition.

References

1. Beysen D, De Paepe A, De Baere E. FOXL2 mutations and genomic rearrangements in BPES. *Hum Mutat.* 2009;30(2):158-169.
2. Anderson RL, Nowinski TS. The five-flap technique for blepharophimosis. *Arch Ophthalmol.* 1989;107(3):448-452.

FINANCIAL DISCLOSURES

Dr. Javaneh Abbasian has no financial or proprietary interest in the materials presented herein.

Dr. Ismael Al Ghamdi has not disclosed any relevant financial relationships.

Dr. Robert W. Arnold is President and board member of Glacier Medical Software, Inc, producer of NICU screening software, ROP-Check. The Alaska Blind Child Discovery (ABCD) has received discounted vision screen technology from several vendors and has received two unrestricted grants from Walmart-Alaska. Dr. Arnold has been an investigator and a paid protocol developer for the Pediatric Eye Disease Investigator Group (PEDIG).

Kyle Arnoldi is supported by an unrestricted grant from Research to Prevent Blindness, New York, New York.

Dr. Nicholas R. Binder has no financial or proprietary interest in the materials presented herein.

Dr. Kara Cavuoto has no financial or proprietary interest in the materials presented herein.

Dr. R.V. Paul Chan has no financial or proprietary interest in the materials presented herein.

Dr. David S. Chu has not disclosed any relevant financial relationships.

Dr. William Constad has no financial or proprietary interest in the materials presented herein.

Dr. Patrick A. DeRespinis has no financial or proprietary interest in the materials presented herein.

Dr. Mark Dorfman has not disclosed any relevant financial relationships.

Dr. Dawn Duss has no financial or proprietary interest in the materials presented herein.

Dr. Brian J. Forbes has no financial or proprietary interest in the materials presented herein.

Dr. Larry Frohman has no financial or proprietary interest in the materials presented herein.

Dr. Florin Grigorian has no financial or proprietary interest in the materials presented herein.

Dr. Paula Grigorian has no financial or proprietary interest in the materials presented herein.

Dr. Suqin Guo has no financial or proprietary interest in the materials presented herein.

Dr. Sheryl M. Handler has no financial or proprietary interest in the materials presented herein.

Dr. Denise Hug has no financial or proprietary interest in the materials presented herein.

Dr. William R. Katowitz has no financial or proprietary interest in the materials presented herein.

Dr. Albert S. Khouri has no financial or proprietary interest in the materials presented herein.

Dr. Paul D. Langer has no financial or proprietary interest in the materials presented herein.

Dr. Steven J. Lichtenstein is a consultant for Alcon Laboratories, Inc.

Dr. Renelle Pointdujour Lim has not disclosed any relevant financial relationships.

Dr. Robert W. Lingua has no financial or proprietary interest in the materials presented herein.

Dr. William Madigan has no financial or proprietary interest in the materials presented herein.

Dr. María Ana Martínez-Castellanos has no financial or proprietary interest in the materials presented herein.

Dr. Linda Nakanishi has no financial or proprietary interest in the materials presented herein.

Dr. Leonard B. Nelson has not disclosed any relevant financial relationships.

Dr. Nina Ni has no financial or proprietary interest in the materials presented herein.

Dr. Christina M. Ohnsman has received lecture fees from Alcon Laboratories, Inc.

Dr. Scott E. Olitsky has no financial or proprietary interest in the materials presented herein.

Dr. Catherine A. Origlieri has no financial or proprietary interest in the materials presented herein.

Dr. Nicole Pritz has no financial or proprietary interest in the materials presented herein.

Dr. Luke Rebenitsch has no financial or proprietary interest in the materials presented herein.

Dr. Ronald Rescigno has no financial or proprietary interest in the materials presented herein.

Dr. Dorothy J. Reynolds has no financial or proprietary interest in the materials presented herein.

Dr. James Reynolds has no financial or proprietary interest in the materials presented herein.

Dr. Carol L. Shields has not disclosed any relevant financial relationships.

Dr. Roman Shinder has no financial or proprietary interest in the materials presented herein.

Dr. Melissa A. Simon has no financial or proprietary interest in the materials presented herein.

Dr. Jonathan C. Song has no financial or proprietary interest in the materials presented herein.

Dr. Roger E. Turbin has not disclosed any relevant financial relationships.

Dr. Rudolph S. Wagner has not disclosed any relevant financial relationships.

INDEX